~~~~~~

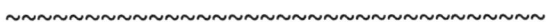

For Mom, who was always in my corner
and for Joan, who always shows up
for the hard parts.

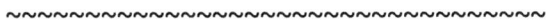

~~~~~~

Table of Contents

How to Use this Book

I wrote this book to collect the information that I found while researching treatments for my mom's cancer care. As a physical therapist, I was well-accustomed to finding peer-reviewed sources of evidence to support my own physical therapy practice, teaching, and research. At the same time, my specialization is not in oncology and so I initially found myself struggling with using the right combination of search terms. I also did not know what I did not know; some newer cancer treatments were not on my radar. I spent a great deal of time when my mom was first diagnosed educating myself so that I could find the information I needed and understand what was relevant to my mom's cancer care.

After my mom's diagnosis, I knew several other people with loved ones who were diagnosed with cancer. I would send them resources and then think of other things I forgot and send a follow up email. I worried that my information wasn't well organized and at the same time overwhelming. At one point, my uncle told me I should write a book and so this project was born.

This book is not an exhaustive guide to cancer and is not meant to replace advice by your healthcare providers. For starters, each type of cancer has different types of treatment that are more effective. Your own biology will also determine what treatments might be better. I have referenced many peer-reviewed published studies that are in the reference section and mention books written for a non-medical audience that I read that aided in my research. Those books are listed separately as resources after the epilogue. I intentionally kept the chapters and the overall length of the book short so that you could quickly find some information that would allow you to hit the ground running. In short, I wanted to save you the time that I lost getting up to speed in the world of cancer.

You can read this book straight through, or you can read the chapters out of order as your needs arise. If you are going to read these out of order would recommend reading Chapter 1 first and then possibly chapter 5 to give you a head start on the diagnosis and second opinions.

Chapter 1 Make Deliberate Early Decisions

It was the fall of 2017 when my mom had a diagnostic ultrasound for gallbladder symptoms. The ultrasound showed sludge in her gallbladder, but also showed a suspicious, hypoechoic area in the pancreas. My mom's father had died from pancreatic cancer when I was a child, so my mom was quickly scheduled for a PET scan. My brother tried to talk me out of my anxiety, but as a physical therapist, I knew that hypoechoic areas on ultrasounds were typically tumors.

I received the call from my mom while I was a work. The PET scan lit up areas in her pancreas. She emailed me her report as I drove home. When I arrived home and read the report, it also mentioned areas of increased uptake in the liver and lung. Regardless of what type of cancer my mom had, there were indications of uptake in multiple organs, it was stage IV.

Living in a large metropolitan area meant that we had many major hospitals from which to choose. We chose based on a great deal of advertising from one of our hospitals, and a few people we knew having positive outcomes for entirely different cancers. This was our first mistake. Just because a hospital is good at treating one type of cancer, does not mean it is good at treating all types of cancer.

Because many of the people we knew with pancreatic cancer had died in days to months from the disease, we rushed this decision. In retrospect, our rushed decision-making cost us valuable time. But, when you hear the words "you have cancer," it seems like you have a ticking time bomb within you ready to detonate and that something needs to be done immediately.

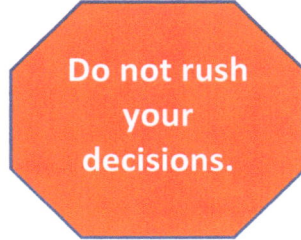

Do not rush your decisions.

We proceeded to that first appointment expecting to see a physician recommended to us. When my mom had called, she had requested an appointment with that physician. We were met by a different doctor. The doctor did not tell us if she was an oncologist or a gastrointestinal doctor. Later, I would google her and find that she was an oncologist. She seemed kind and caring. She explained that she believed my mom had cancer and that it had started in her pancreas. She said she would like their radiologist to read my mom's PET scan images to make sure that they were read properly. She also wanted my mom to have some bloodwork to test for the cancer marker CA 19-9, which when elevated beyond 200, typically indicates pancreatic cancer. The doctor spent a lot of time with us and we felt comfortable with her.

My mom and I cried and clung to each other in the waiting room, while we sat listening for her name to be called for her bloodwork. I texted my husband after they took my mom back. We made a follow-up appointment for the next week. As we waited for our cars from the valet, I told my mom I would do anything I could to help save her life. This started our journey towards gathering information and was the first step in regaining control.

I really didn't sleep much over that intervening week. My mind turned over all sorts of worries and regrets. My older daughter was the age I was when my mom's father died. I remembered how hard that year was for me- both the weeks he lived with his diagnosis and the aftermath. I thought of all of the things my daughters did with my mom-snowboarding, going to the beach, baking. My mom was the grandmother everyone dreams of having. She even helped homeschool my daughter and so I also felt pressure to have a backup plan, without making it seem like I was giving up on my mom. There were trips we had postponed until my dad's health improved. Would we ever get to go?

Finally, the follow-up appointment arrived. The doctor told us that my mom's CA 19-9 was 48,000 (remember >200 was diagnostic of pancreatic cancer). She said my mom could not delay in starting chemotherapy. They would do a liver biopsy and place a port for chemo simultaneously. The doctor referred my mom to genetic testing as that would drive the treatment selection if my mom was a BRCA carrier, which are inherited mutations that can cause cancers in the breast, ovaries, and pancreas. We asked about their radiologist reading the PET scan and the doctor told us that it wasn't necessary, despite her recommending that at the prior appointment. The doctor would not give us an answer as to why this was no longer necessary. We asked about an endoscopic ultrasound with biopsy of the pancreas, and she said that wasn't necessary either. I have since learned that this is a recommended procedure with a pancreatic cancer diagnosis. My mom expressed the desire to wait to start chemotherapy until after Christmas. The doctor was upset with my mom and told her that with a delay in treatment, my mom could be dead within months. I had a feeling that we were being rushed into treatment and that the doctor no longer had time for us.

My mom and I left with instructions that the biopsy and genetic testing appointment would be scheduled. My mom carried her cell phone with her everywhere to make sure she didn't miss the phone call. While genetic testing was scheduled quickly, no phone call came for the biopsy and port placement. My mom called several times and finally scheduling called back. The only available time they had was three weeks away. We spoke with scheduling about how urgently the oncologist had wanted my mom to start chemotherapy, but we were told that this was the only day available.

By now, I was panicking due to the lack of communication from this hospital. I told my mom we needed a second opinion. We scheduled an appointment towards the end of January at another major hospital an hour and a half away that had a top-rated pancreatic cancer center. In the meantime, my mom was given the link to a video to watch about chemo from the original hospital. There was no meeting with the doctor to discuss chemotherapy options or rationale for one treatment over another. When my mom called the doctor to point out that she hadn't done genetic testing yet, the doctor told her, "It isn't necessary. We know what it is."

We went through with the genetic testing at that hospital since it was scheduled. The genetic counselor was kind and answered all of our questions, such as how different mutations could positively impact treatment or negatively impact prognosis and if my brother and I should undergo genetic testing if my mom was positive for a mutation. She showed us how she sketched out the family tree as she asked my mom questions pertaining to her family health history. She told my mom she would call with results in two weeks after explaining what genetic markers she was looking for including BRCA and how that could help guide treatment and improve survival rates.

After this, my mom went for her liver biopsy and port placement. My brother accompanied her as I was giving a final exam that day. I was so glad that he was there to advocate for her and take notes. Despite previously being told otherwise, they were informed upon arrival that they never place a port on the same day as a liver biopsy as it was too dangerous. My mom said the doctor performing the procedure had challenges finding her tumors and one of the nurses in the room was providing different suggestions to the doctor, including trying a different machine. This did not foster confidence. After my mom came home, she promptly cancelled the rescheduled port placement and chemotherapy at that hospital.

We scheduled an appointment with a local hospital the day after Christmas so that we had an option closer to home. This appointment went so much better. The pancreas surgeon told my mom that at present she was not a surgical candidate, but that if she were his sister, he would tell his sister to pursue chemotherapy. We had ourselves a good cry and the oncology nurse gave us time to pull ourselves together. She even tried to get us a same-day appointment with the oncologist. He was on vacation but agreed to come back a day early so that she could have an appointment the following day. We were relieved with this efficiency and compassion. At that appointment the next day, the oncologist said he felt it was necessary for my mom to undergo an endoscopic ultrasound with a pancreas biopsy to confirm that my mom truly had cancer and that it had indeed started in the pancreas. He said the liver biopsy my mom had was a fine needle aspiration versus a core biopsy. The fine needle aspiration did not always provide a good sample.

We scheduled the endoscopic ultrasound quickly. My mom's sister took my mom to the appointment and I met my aunt there. We nervously sat together while we waited for my mom to be brought into the recovery room. Finally, they called us back. When my mom was fully awake, the doctor who had performed the procedure came to her bedside to explain that she did have pancreatic cancer with metastases to her liver. The official diagnosis was stage IV mucinous adenocarcinoma of the pancreas. They had managed to get a tissue sample of the pancreas tumor that could be used for molecular typing. The doctor and the nurses gave my mom a card they had all signed wishing her strength and healing. This simple gesture relieved a little of the burden we had been handed.

We met with the oncologist again and he suggested my mom consider either a clinical trial they were running or starting Folfirinox – a three-drug chemotherapy regimen that is a first line treatment of pancreatic cancer. We met with the nurse in charge of the clinical trial and listened to the study protocol. My mom asked if she would be able to skip a week of chemo to go on a trip we were trying to plan. The nurse explained that because this was a clinical trial, the protocol had to be followed precisely. My mom thanked her for her time but declined treatment in the study. My mom had her life to live. She wanted to include holistic treatment as well (discussed in chapter 6), which was another aspect forbidden by a clinical trial. The doctor came back to explain that Folfirinox would be an infusion of Oxaliplatin and Irinotecan followed by being sent home with a 48-hour pump of 5-FU in a fanny pack. He said my mom could do her daily activities while on the pump. He did not; however, ask what her daily activities were. We did not think to ask what he had in mind regarding daily activities; we knew what my mom's daily activities were and so we just accepted that at face value. My mom was set up for port placement. The doctor encouraged her to keep the appointment at what was supposed to be her second opinion so that she was in that hospital's system in case a clinical trial opened up for which she was eligible. The geneticist called as we were leaving the appointment and stated no genetic markers for pancreatic cancer were found. At that point, we closed out our time with that first hospital, although my mom continued to get mailings from them regarding neuroendocrine tumors of the pancreas – which was not the type of cancer she had.

We drove the 90 minutes and stayed overnight at a hotel to be ready for the early appointment at what was now a third opinion. The doctor agreed with Folfirinox as the first line of treatment. He told my mom that the first hospital had yet to send the tissue sample six weeks after the initial request. He explained that they did know from reports that she was microsatellite stable; microsatellite instability is a change in the genetic code of a tumor which provides additional treatment options. We left feeling discouraged but knowing that the treatment that my mom was slated to start at the second hospital was the appropriate choice. At this point, I began to research both traditional and holistic treatment options.

My mom went in for her port placement. My aunt and I went to the first chemotherapy appointment just in case my mom didn't feel well enough to drive home. My aunt was planning on staying with my mom for the weekend so that she wasn't alone. My mom's CA 19-9 had increased to 100,000. We were worried that the delay in treatment resulted in an elevation in my mom's tumor markers. My mom tolerated the chemo treatment well in the office but was sent home with a big purse-like pump for the 5-FU. My mom asked if she could run or ski with the pump and was told no, the danger of pulling out the infusion was too high and if she did that, toxic chemicals would leak out. So much for doing her daily activities. My mom had a terrible weekend of nausea and flu-like symptoms and lost several pounds. When she came back for the next infusion, they decided to eliminate the Irinotecan as the nurse felt that was what had made my mom so sick. The nurse commented that a lot of people don't come back for more than one treatment because the chemo makes them so sick.

My mom's cousin is a functional medicine doctor in California and had looked into holistic care. Simultaneously, I was doing the same thing. Both of us turned up the Berkson protocol,[1-3] which consisted of IV infusions of Vitamin C and Alpha Lipoic Acid (ALA). We both felt like this was a sign to pursue this holistic treatment in addition to chemotherapy. I started investigating local physicians that did infusions.

So now we had a plan for both chemotherapy and a framework for holistic care. This plan evolved over time. The roots of that evolution are interwoven in the following chapter.

A Note about Deliberate Decisions

The deliberate decisions you make today, may lead you to make new deliberate decisions in 3 months, 6 months, a year or more after diagnosis. New research about your type of cancer might come out, or a new drug might be approved for your cancer. You might decide to change oncologists or add another member to your healthcare team. Your decisions now do not rule out a change of treatment or provider later. Keep an open mind on your journey.

❖❖❖❖❖❖❖❖❖❖❖❖❖❖❖❖❖
Notes and Questions
❖❖❖❖❖❖❖❖❖❖❖❖❖❖❖❖❖

Chapter 2 Make Social Connections

You may have a variety of reactions to being told you have cancer. You might reach out to a few loved ones or close friends to get support. Some people might go onto the internet or social media to search for online support. Others might post an announcement to social media to rally people around them. There is no correct way to respond to the news that you have cancer. My mom and I are both very private people. When my mom learned that she had cancer, she did not want to tell anyone other than close family and a few friends. This was challenging for me because many of her friends had children with whom I was close friends. It would put everyone in a difficult spot if I reached out to friends for support and their parents didn't know. What if a friend slipped up and mentioned the cancer to their parents? I had to sit down and explain to my mom that as a caregiver, I needed a support network so that I could care for her while staying mentally healthy and focused for her. My mom eventually relented and let me know which of her friends knew that she had cancer. For the duration of her life, it remained a small number of people and caused a bit of tension, but I respected her privacy.

That said, casting a wide social net regarding cancer can be of great benefit. My mom told one of her closest friends from her working days; that friend's relative reached out to me with advice on questions that I needed to be asking any physician with whom we connected. Her husband also had a pancreas tumor, albeit a different type, and this advice helped me realize that the second opinion was needed as soon as possible.

I reached out to a friend of mine living in Boston. A close friend of hers Jennifer* had lived with stage IV pancreatic cancer for years and I wanted to know what tips she had. My friend connected the two of us and we spent the better part of an hour talking about both holistic and conventional treatment options, as well as promising clinical trials we should investigate. I checked in with Jennifer periodically and she gave me both updates on her health and advice for my mom. We eventually met with Jennifer's oncologist in Boston, two years later, as he was creative in his treatment approach and we felt we needed creative thinking at that point. We left that appointment with hope and a more cohesive plan than we had in place.

A week or two after my mom's initial diagnosis, I broke down sobbing while getting my haircut. It was the first chance I had to breathe in several weeks and I think just taking that time for myself caused me to open the floodgates. My stylist was very nice, bringing me tissues and water. She also brought me to the front desk to talk to the salon owner, whose best friend had stage IV breast cancer. She talked me through different homeopathic options, took my email down and sent me about 20 resources by the end of the day. Most importantly, she connected me with a local integrative doctor who only worked with patients with cancer. We called this physician and set up an appointment for the first available day they had. From that point on, any time the salon owner or I found new information for cancer supportive care, we emailed it to the other person in an attempt to help each other.

While at my daughters' Nutcracker ballet dress rehearsal, I mentioned to the studio owner's mother that my mother was diagnosed with cancer. She pointed me to several holistic options, including the Gerson protocol. She also directed me to the

New York Times "War on Cancer"
www.cancerdecisions.com
by
Ralph Moss, PhD

website www.cancerdecisions.com by Ralph Moss, PhD, who wrote the New York Times "War on Cancer" column for many years.[1] For a few hundred dollars, you could purchase a synthesized report on evidence for both conventional and holistic treatment. This was one of the best purchases that we made for a few reasons. The first was that providing me with the names of various holistic treatment options allowed me to run PubMed.gov searches on further evidence for these treatments and potential side effects. Pubmed is an online database of published medical and life science articles and books. This assisted me in focusing my PubMed searches instead of blindly performing general searches of holistic care and cancer. The Moss report also rates the treatments as green light-meaning they were

	Red light meaning the treatment was not safe and/or not effective
	Yellow light meaning that safety and/or efficacy hadn't been established
	Green light meaning safe and had good evidence supporting their use

safe and had good evidence supporting their use, yellow light meaning that safety and/or efficacy hadn't been established and red light meaning the treatment was not safe and/or not effective.

As a result of these initial social connections, we met with the integrative doctor. He recommended various supplements as well as mistletoe injections; mistletoe extract can help to stimulate the immune system. He also presented us with the Berkson protocol that I mentioned in the prior chapter.[2-4]

He worked with my mom and I to start a regimen of initial supplements (my mom did not want to give herself injections) and I found a doctor willing to infuse vitamin C and ALA. By the beginning of March, holistic care was added to my mom's treatment plan.

Social connections are not just important for finding cancer treatment options. Research demonstrates that social connections have a bearing on our health. In fact, Dr. Kelly Turner's research into radial remission has found that social support is one of the key factors in people who have experienced a radical remission.[5] Cultivating and maintaining social connections is critical to health and longevity even in the absence of a cancer diagnosis.

Social Support Networks and Health Outcomes for Patients and Caregivers

Social support may be somewhat dependent on the quality of your relationships. When we consider social networks, this is the set of relationships that you participate in and can consist of friends, family members, colleagues, members of other groups you belong to such as your religious community, your book club, or your running group. Support comes in different forms. There is the general support we received from the relationships we have whether they are familial, romantic, or friendship. There is also functional or structural support which involves caregiving tasks like cooking, cleaning and taking a loved one to doctor appointments.

Some structural ties might be stronger than others.[6,7] The strength of a tie of a social support is measured by the length of time the people involved know each other and the intensity of the relationship. A work acquaintance you have known for two years versus your best friend 40 years are going to have different strength values. Having a diverse social support network could provide you with a greater influx of information and ideas; a social support network that has friends from different stages of your life, co-workers, from places like your religious institution, as well as family members may help to provide you with a broader range of information. These wider networks of more complex social ties have less density, because those people do not necessarily know each other. However, this does allow for a multitude of perspectives. Those multitude of perspectives may provide you with some new information related to your diagnosis. I certainly saw that in my own case as I reached out to diverse people, whether it was my daughters' ballet studio, my physical therapy colleagues, or my own family members. Having a large social network with people from various areas of your life that you are frequently in contact with is associated with a reduction in mortality for people with chronic diseases such as cancer over a 15-year period.[8] Regardless of how dense your social network is, your primary social support network is whoever you can rely on the most. You may feel reluctant to burden your primary social support network; however, evidence suggests that caregivers in stronger, higher-quality relationships experience lower levels of perceived caregiver burden.[9]

Social support can mediate the stress response in your body, which in turn has a mediating effect on inflammation. Inflammation is associated both with cancer diagnosis and outcomes. [10] One smaller study found that female breast cancer survivors who perceived they had a stronger social support network had decreased measures of reactivity in the amygdala, which is the area of the brain responsible for processing emotions including fear and anxiety.[10] The women also had decreased inflammatory markers such as C-reactive protein and IL-6. In addition to stress and inflammation, social support, hope, and resilience are all significantly and positively associated with quality of life, with social support having the strongest association. [11] This is not surprising since social support mediates depression and anxiety symptoms. [12,13] For patients with advanced cancer, one thing that helps to reduce depressive symptoms is having positive relationships with their loved ones. Advanced cancer is often associated with increased burden of symptoms and a simultaneous rise in anxiety and demoralization. Strong social connections help to reduce the demoralization that people with advanced cancer experience.[14]

Social support and education of caregivers can improve both the physical and mental wellbeing of both the caregiver and the patient.[15] Social support and easing caregiver burden are critical both in preventing caregiver burnout and in improving the health of the patient. Social support for caregivers is critical to improve their own well-being and can also influence the health and well-being of the person receiving the care.[16]

Having strong, positive social interactions with and experiencing affection from a support system is important for each of us, but particularly when facing a diagnosis such as cancer.[17] Perceiving that you are receiving sufficient social support is associated with decreased need for a referral to psychological services.[18] Having a network who is interested in listening to you about your cancer and your concerns is important to your well-being.[19] This might be family and friends but could also come from a cancer-specific support group. People with cancer sometimes note that their close family and friends may either be overprotective or distant, making it hard to get the right kind of support.[19] It is important that you find a social support network that can meet your needs. If your close family cannot hear your concerns because their own worries make it hard for them to listen, then you will need to look beyond them for this kind of support.

Some patients feel that their cancer diagnosis has a silver lining. Your social support network can help you talk through and process your cancer diagnosis and help you focus on the positive.[20] Maybe you have discovered a genetic component to your cancer and your family members are getting screened. Maybe you reconnected with an estranged family member as the result of your diagnosis. While it is good to focus on positive emotions, the ability to express and accept the range of emotions surrounding your diagnosis and acceptance of the diagnosis is important.[20] Women in one study found that experiencing love and support from other people allowed them to understand who their true friends were, and helped bring their families closer together.[20] This study finding is interesting to me because we personally found that our social support network was much wider than we had anticipated. My mom stated that she did not understand why so many people were helping her and that she had never felt so loved in her entire life. I think we both benefitted from the phone calls, texts, emails and visits with friends and family; we felt support as our social connections rallied around us. Evidence suggests that finding the silver lining in your cancer diagnosis can reduce depressive symptoms through fostering acceptance your diagnosis and the emotions that come with it, while eliciting and strengthening positive responses from a social network.[20]

Social support can be useful in helping people develop self-efficacy, or their belief in themselves to take charge of their health.[21]

When patients with cancer perceive strong social support, it can lead to a greater belief that they could take care of themselves and their illness. One potential source of support for somebody who is uncomfortable reaching out to friends and family is a peer support network. Peer support is an intentionally designed support network in which a person who has undergone the same experiences - in this case cancer - would help to provide emotional support, empathy and understanding of the situation from a personal level. Peer support networks can share information related to a specific diagnosis, provide affirmations or supportive statements, and can help them problem solve.[22]

We know that the larger a person's social network is the lower mortality; having a strong social network actually helps to promote longevity.[23] A social network, and in particular the spouse or partner, that provides support at the time of diagnosis can help to provide social support, allow for the development and reinforcement of coping skills ,and may help to obtain additional information about a cancer diagnosis.[24] One study examined over 9000 women who had had breast cancer. [7] Women who had stronger social support networks had reduced risk for mortality from both breast cancer- and non-breast cancer-related causes. Additionally, women who were socially isolated had a stronger risk of recurrence than those who had stronger social support networks. Social isolation and reduced support are in fact associated with increased mortality across a range of cancer diagnoses.[25] Men diagnosed with prostate cancer who live alone have a higher risk of dying from the disease, but this risk can be decreased by increasing connections through social activities. [26] Social isolation is also associated with moderate-to-high fear of recurrence, which can impact quality of life and well-being even in the absence of cancer.[27]

Depression often accompanies a cancer diagnosis. One study examined African American women with a diagnosis of breast cancer. Those who were married, who had a higher degree of spirituality, and who had lower depressive symptoms perceived a greater amount of social support.[28] However, women who experienced a decline in social support in the year post diagnosis experienced an increase in depressive symptoms and had lower self-ratings of their own health.

Emotional distress and depression increase as social support declines in the year post treatment for breast cancer.[29] This relationship; however, only holds true if you look at the quantity of social support. A higher quality of the social support received supports emotional well-being in women post-treatment, lending further support to the idea that the number of your connections is not as important as the type of support being received. Having a few key people that you can rely on may be more important than having a variety of people who come to the forefront after your diagnosis, but then fade into the background as your treatment continues. Density and strength of social support network (structural support) as well as total support are associated with decreased risk of disease progression, and support through caregiver tasks (functional support), is also associated with this to a lesser extent.[30] In other words, stronger but fewer ties is better for your mental and physical health than a multitude of weaker ties.

Receiving a cancer diagnosis can cause a great deal of distress. Distress can be due to a decline in health and physical function. Instrumental support helps alleviate the distress from decline in function in people actively undergoing treatment; emotional support can alleviate this distress in those who have completed treatment. Social support has a greater impact in alleviating distress in people with the greatest physical decline.[31]

The relationship between stress, social support, and cancer mortality is not to be underestimated. One Swedish study looked at men with prostate cancer.[32] The study examined perceived stress in men diagnosed with prostate cancer, as well as their social support network. Living alone was associated with increased risk of mortality, whereas the men who engaged in a greater number of social activities had lower mortality. Engaging in social activities as best as you are able to participate may improve your lifespan. Identify a few areas in which you can socialize. If you are experiencing fatigue this could be face-timing with a friend or watching a movie with friends or family. If you have more energy, be sure to get out and do something fun with your friends and family.

Increased mortality is also associated with increased rates of perceived stress.[32] Higher levels of perceived stress are associated with higher frequencies of sleep loss;[32] the relationship between sleep and wellness is critical. Getting enough sleep will help promote wellness. Higher perceived stress may be due to lower social support networks or an inability to share distress and concerns with a social support network.[32] This emphasizes the need to seek out a formal peer support network if you are uncomfortable sharing your concerns with your loved ones. However, please realize that your social support network is there for you not just in good times but also in hard times. Reach out to your friends and family. You may even have different friends and family members you reach out to for different concerns.

If you have completed your cancer treatments, social connections are still important. Many people complete treatment but still experience a fear of cancer returning. In some respects, low levels of this fear will help you remain vigilant about cancer screenings and keeping your medical appointments. However, high levels of fear of recurrence could in fact end up causing debilitating anxiety. Social connectedness can help reduce fear of disease recurrence, as social isolation is associated with this fear.[27] Maintaining your social connections improves longevity and can reduce the fear of cancer returning to lower, more acceptable levels once you have completed cancer treatment.

Online Social Support

Social support doesn't just have to be face-to-face social support, it could also be virtual. Social media, such as Facebook can be used to communicate about cancer.[33,34] Social media can raise awareness about a specific cancer or to help gain support for caregivers. But people also use Facebook to document their journey, to share their own emotional distress, and to gain emotional support as well as to express gratitude for that support. Because cancer treatments can be costly, Facebook can help fundraise to defray the costs of care.[33,34] You may feel unwilling to ask for this type of support, but often friends and family are willing to contribute when made aware of how costly cancer treatment is.

Social support via online forums can be for exchanging information, for encouragement, or for tangible assistance such as finding grants to pay for treatment or locating relevant clinical trials.[35] One app that I found useful during my mom's illness was the Belong app, which provides disease-specific support forums where you can exchange information and receive emotional support from other patients and their caregivers going through the same disease process.[36] It also has forums for disease-specific information where you could ask an oncologist questions related to specific treatments or where you could receive clinical trial information. This app was helpful for us as there was vetted health information from healthcare providers as well as just that exchange of information and emotional support from other people going through the same treatment. Online forums may be particularly useful as people who are undergoing cancer treatment and who may not have the energy to go to face-to-face support groups.[35] Thus, the internet can be an excellent support group for those too tired to attend support groups.

Likewise, caregivers may not have the time to attend face-to-face support groups.[35] Caregivers who are pressed for time may find the convenience of online support valuable. As a caregiver, you might find that online support helps you as a caregiver to receive support in order to promote your own mental health and wellbeing, while providing you with information that you might need to more quickly be able to assist your loved one. Online interventions for caregivers can improve caregivers' self-efficacy, perceived social support and reduce emotional burden.[37]

There are certainly many different ways that both patients and caregivers participate in online support groups. Some people are more vested and participate a great deal, possibly due to a longer time since diagnosis or a higher stage of cancer.[35] At the other end of the spectrum are people who lurk and just read comments without direct participation. It can be problematic when a small percentage of people contribute most of the content, leaving the unheard majority of people in these forums to potentially not benefit from this type of support.[35] It may be that the communication rendered in these forums might discourage others to participate. For example, in the case of my mother's diagnosis of pancreatic cancer there were sometimes people who were very negative in disease-specific forums. It could be challenging for people who were still trying to cure their cancer or have no evidence of disease (NED) on their scans to see comments from others being very negative about the loss of their loved ones in the same forum. Additionally, people may cease participating or drop out completely from a group. You might find groups that you initially joined to gain information, no longer serve their purpose. I was in one Facebook group to help to get information regarding a specific holistic approach to support my mom, but I found that moderators would only approve certain types of questions, leaving me to research these answers on my own. I do think it is important that you join a variety of online forums, and then find the ones that have evidence-based information on either allopathic or complementary medicine.(Table 2.1) The key is to find groups that provide you the information you are looking for, while providing support that is positive and encouraging, and allows for a multitude of opinions.

Table 2.1 Levels of Evidence from Highest to Lowest

Systematic reviews and meta-analyses	A study that combines the results of multiple studies to find out the overall effect of a treatment or other intervention such as exercise
Randomized controlled trial	A clinical trial in which participants are randomly assigned to the treatment group or to the control group. In clinical trials involving cancer, the control is typically the standard medication provided for that particular type of cancer.
Cohort Studies	These are studies that follow people and record their natural exposure to factors that can increase or decrease their risk for developing certain diseases. The factors can be things such as environmental pollutants, dietary choices and exercise. Development of disease in people who were and were not exposed to the factor of interest is compared to see if the factor increased or decreased the risk for developing a disease.

Table 2.1 continued

Case-control study	These studies look at people who have a disease and compare them to people who do not have the disease. Factors that might increase or decrease the chances of developing the disease are examined retrospectively to see if there is an association between these factors and developing the disease.
Case series or case studies	These studies describe a disease or treatment process in one or a few patients with the same diagnosis.
Expert opinion	These are opinions grounded in science and based upon a person's clinical experience.
Newspaper or magazine articles	These articles often cite scientific journal articles as sources. It is always best to go back and read the original article to make sure the journalist's interpretation of the findings is accurate.
Blogs and personal webpages	These have varying accuracy. If the writer has a strong background in medicine or science, this could be a credible source of evidence. It is always best to do further research to make sure that information posted in a blog has research behind it.

Getting Specific Support

Caregivers need to stay healthy to support their loved one with cancer and people with cancer need support in order to focus on getting well. Needing help and not receiving it can negatively impact health. Sometimes loved ones want to help and may not know how to help. Sometimes loved ones try to help you in ways that are really not what is needed. If your loved ones have not come up with a list of specific ways they can help you, tell them the things that you need help with, whether it is meals, or somebody to come to doctor's appointments to help take notes and ask questions, or somebody to vent about your frustration with your disease. (Box 2.1) Anything you can think of in terms of your needs is important to you and can help your support network divide up tasks.

Many caregivers find that their relationships with their loved one improve within these caregiver tasks.[39] I myself found a great deal of privilege in helping to make meals for my mom. This is something she would not ordinarily let me do. But I enjoy cooking and I show my love through gifts of food. For me, this was a way that I could make sure that she was having nutritionally balanced meals while taking one task off of her plate. Our tastes in food are quite different, so I had to make sure I was making meals she would eat and I learned a lot about her food preferences in the process. She also expanded the foods she would eat. We both found joy and meaning in that.

Box 2.1 Suggestions for Caregiver Tasks

- Checking in via call, email or text
- Listening
- Supporting your loved one in their treatment decisions
- Be a sounding board for treatment options
- Taking loved one out, for example to eat or to the movies
- Making meals
- Cleaning
- Food shopping
- Making appointments
- Driving to appointments
- Finding potential healthcare practitioners
- Researching different treatment options
- Taking notes at appointments
- Childcare for your loved one's child(ren)
- Driving child(ren) to activities
- Making playdates
- Performing yardwork
- Addressing home repairs
- Picking up medications

Caregiver Support and Cancer Care

One thing to remember when we're thinking about social support is that support related to cancer decision-making may or may not be desired from the loved ones with cancer. If you are a caregiver, be respectful about the amount of support that your loved one might desire. If you are living with cancer, communicate clearly about your needs. One area in which this is particularly beneficial is with respect to decision-making regarding cancer treatment options.

Every individual has their own style of decision making, which might mean that caregivers and loved ones have a mismatch of style. One recent study focused on cancer treatment, decision making and how patients and families work together or arrive at decisions separately with respect to cancer treatment.[40] As caregivers, we need to consider different types of decision making (Table 2.2).

Caregivers should be mindful of serving their loved ones in the manner that it is needed. Providing more support than is needed can reinforce the sick role in your loved one and can create a feeling of helplessness or decreased self-efficacy.[31] While we want to help our loved ones, we don't want to make them feel dependent. Asking a loved one what type of help they would like is important. A caregiver might say something along the lines of, "I would like to be a partner in your decision making. Would you like or need that? Who else would you like to be involved in your decision-making process?" This gives a starting point for a conversation in which caregivers do not take control over a situation that ultimately isn't theirs, while also creating a framework of a support network to which tasks can be delegated. This is not the same thing as saying, 'how can I help?' which is vague. By saying, "I would like to help you and I have come up with a list of ways that I think I might be of help. Please let me know if any of these things would be useful for you, so that you can focus on your health and I can take some of the load from you. Please let me know if there are any other ways I can help you that I didn't identify on my list." It may be that a loved one falls into that independent category and does not want help or input, or it may be that they identify something that was not placed on the original list and a caregiver might not particularly want to do. However, if a caregiver offers help and it isn't wanted, the caregiver needs to accept this, as this is the most loving and supportive thing you can do. If a caregiver offers help and a different need is identified, then the caregiver needs to be willing to do this, as this is the help that is needed.

Table 2.2 Types of Decision Making[40]

Type	Definition
Isolated	• Desires help and support, but does not receive any
Collaborative	• Interdependent type of decision-making, loved ones are invited to share in the decision making • Patient chooses how much of the decision making is performed by the family
Delegated	• Patient turns over decision making to their family
Demeaning	• Patient has no desired support for decision making, but receives support anyway
Independent	• Patient does not desire and does not receive support

Another recent study looked at decision-making styles in patients with cancer and whether or not they wanted to collaborate and have social support in their cancer decision-making.[41] The majority of participants surveyed felt that they received the most social and decision-making support from their oncologist, followed by a significant other/spouse. The older adults in the study felt that they only had support from their oncologist and did not have an issue with that. Even though the older adults were more independent, they also were the most satisfied with their decision-making collaboration with their oncologists. Additionally, people in this study who had higher socioeconomic status reported that they had greater levels of satisfaction in collaboration with their oncologists.[41] This finding might indicate that patients with greater economic resources are more empowered and better able to make a wider range of decisions. People with greater resources also may be less deferential to their oncologist or may have a wider choice in oncologist based on health insurance, allowing for greater satisfaction in that collaboration. Even if health insurance requires the use of a particular oncologist, patients still have a right to be in collaboration and receive support from another oncologist.

So, if you are someone living with cancer, identify and reach out to your social network. Tell them what specific needs you might have. Ask questions and expect support and answers from your oncologist. If you are not receiving this from your oncologist, seek another opinion, as you deserve collaboration in your care. If you are a caregiver, be prepared with a list of ways you can help your loved one but remember to seek support for yourself. It isn't helpful to let your own mental and physical health suffer while you support your loved one with cancer.

❖❖❖❖❖❖❖❖❖❖❖❖❖❖❖❖❖❖❖
Notes and Questions
❖❖❖❖❖❖❖❖❖❖❖❖❖❖❖❖❖❖❖

Chapter 3 Cancer Testing and Treatment

After your diagnosis, you may need additional testing and will need to make decisions about cancer treatment based on the results of this testing. You may be overwhelmed with the number of appointments you have and by the medical jargon that is thrown at you. Going into your appointment with information about what testing is typical for your specific type of cancer as well as what general tests are performed for anyone with cancer is helpful. This chapter will cover typical testing that may occur as part of your diagnosis.

My mom's initial cancer diagnosis was based on an ultrasound, followed by a PET scan. She also had a Chest CT, bloodwork, a liver biopsy and an endoscopic ultrasound with pancreas biopsy. This represented six separate appointments for tests that were not explained to my mom. Fortunately, I knew what these tests were and could explain them to my mom. Suddenly, my healthy mom who only went to the doctor once a year for a physical had 6 appointments in a matter of weeks. After the results of these tests, she then had to make a decision as to whether she would enroll in a clinical trial for an experimental chemotherapy drug or have chemotherapy. The clinical trial decision had to be made on the spot, because she needed to not have had any treatment to enroll in that particular clinical trial. My mom declined the clinical trial as it would prevent her from also engaging in holistic treatment, which will be covered in future chapters.

Cancer Staging

Your cancer will need to be staged. Imaging tests such as a CT scan, an MRI, an ultrasound, or a PET scan might be performed. Lab tests such as blood tests can also help to stage some types of cancer. While you may hear people talking about their cancer being stage one or stage four, typically your oncologist will use the TNM system, which varies slightly depending on the type of cancer you have.[1] The T category refers to the primary tumor and is concerned with tumor size, location, and whether it has grown into nearby sites. The T category is typically staged 1 through 4; the higher the T number, the larger the tumor, or the more it's grown into nearby tissues. The N category stands for lymph nodes and is assigned a number between 0-3. A zero means no lymph node involvement; N 1-3 describes the size, location or number of nearby lymph nodes affected by cancer. The higher the N number, the greater the cancer spread to lymph nodes. M stands for metastasis. M0 means there is no metastases and M1 means the cancer has spread to distant organs or tissues, for example my mom's pancreas cancer had spread to her liver. [1] Solid tumors will be staged differently than blood cancers.

Cancer may also be referred to by a numerical stage. (Table 3.1). It is important to note that if your cancer responds to treatment, your cancer will not be restaged. If you were diagnosed at stage 4, even if you reach no evidence of disease (NED), you will still be considered stage 4.

Table 3.1. General Cancer Staging [2]

Cancer Stage	Description
0	• Cancer is in situ, has not spread • Highly curable
1	• Small tumor • Has not grown deeply into nearby tissue • Has not spread to lymph nodes or other parts of the body
2-3	• Larger tumors • Has grown into nearby tissues • May involve lymph nodes
4	• Cancer has spread to other organs or parts of the body • Also called advanced or metastatic cancer

Bloodwork

You may have bloodwork taken. The complete blood count (CBC) is one test that can help to diagnose some cancers, particularly leukemia or lymphoma. [3] Bloodwork can help to see if the cancer has spread to the bone marrow, can determine if side effects of chemotherapy that involve the blood are occurring, and can determine how your body is responding to cancer treatment. A CBC measures white blood cell, red blood cell and platelet counts. The white blood cell count measures the total number of white blood cells in a sample of blood. White blood cells, or leukocytes, are responsible for fighting off infection and can be decreased in response to cancer treatment. The white blood cell differential measures each of the five types of white blood cell. There are five different types of white blood cells. Chemotherapy can lower your white blood cells. You may be given an injection to help to prevent low white cell count. The different types of white blood cells provide information about your health. Having higher number of lymphocytes or monocytes can indicate the presence of certain cancers. Some cancer might deplete or reduce the number of neutrophils, which can make it easier to get a bacterial infection. [3]

Red blood cells, or erythrocytes, carry oxygen throughout your body. Your hematocrit value is the percentage of blood that is made up of red blood cells and the hemoglobin value is the amount of protein in red blood cells that carry oxygen. Having lower hematocrit and hemoglobin can be of concern during cancer treatment. Low red count can indicate anemia, which is one possible side effect of chemo or radiation therapy and is sometimes the result of cancer itself. If your red count falls too low, you might need a blood transfusion or medication to raise it.[3]

Platelets help to clot blood, which is important in wound healing. Some cancer treatments can lower your platelet count. Cancers that involve the bone marrow can also lower your platelet count; multiple myeloma can actually raise your platelet count to abnormal levels. A low platelet count increases your risk of bleeding and bruising. You might need platelet transfusions if your platelet count falls to very low levels.[3]

You may also have tumor marker testing performed on your blood sample.[4] The CA 19-9 test that my mom had was a specific tumor marker test for pancreatic cancer. However, these tests aren't perfect and often are not specific enough. The CA 19-9 test is not specific enough to aid in early diagnosis of pancreatic cancer, for example, and can be elevated from other conditions as well.

There are different tumor marker tests for specific cancers, although many cancers do not have a specific tumor marker test.[4] Depending on how good the tumor marker test is at ruling in or out the presence of cancer, it may be used for different reasons. Some tumor markers can be used to diagnose a specific cancer, some to determine if the cancer treatment is working, and some to even determine if a targeted therapy is appropriate. [5] The National Cancer Institute list of common tumor markers can be found at https://www.cancer.gov/about-cancer/diagnosis-staging/diagnosis/tumor-markers-list. [5]

Biopsies

You might have a biopsy of your tumor if it is a solid tumor, your bone marrow. or your lymph nodes. If you have an entire organ surgically removed, such as a kidney, then the tumor might be biopsied after your surgery.[6] There are two other types of biopsies. Excisional biopsies are where a surgeon removes an entire tumor. These can be performed using minimally invasive surgeries that are guided with a camera such as a laparoscope or thoracoscope. [6] In the case of skin cancer, you may have a biopsy of the skin which will not need imaging or special cameras to view as in the cases of internal cancers. [6] My mom had an endoscopic biopsy, where the camera was introduced into the upper part of the digestive tract, through the esophagus, to where it connected to the stomach. From there, the doctor was able to do an incisional biopsy of the pancreas; this type of biopsy removes part of the tumor for examination in a laboratory.

You might also have a needle biopsy. The first type of needle biopsy is fine needle aspiration in which a syringe attached to a thin, hollow needle is used to take out some fluid and tissue from the tumor. If your tumor is close to the surface of your body, the doctor might feel for the tumor before inserting the needle. The doctor might also use imaging such as ultrasound to see where the needle should be inserted. A core biopsy also uses a syringe, but the needle is larger and removes a cylinder of tissue. Local anesthesia is used to numb the area.[6] My mom had a fine needle aspiration of the tumor of her liver, which was guided by ultrasound.

Lymph nodes may also be biopsied.[6] Sentinel lymph node mapping helps a surgeon know which lymph nodes need to be removed for biopsy and can help your oncologist understand whether cancer has spread to your lymph nodes. To identify which lymph nodes the tumor is draining to, radioactive dye is injected into the tumor. About an hour later, the lymph nodes that the dye traveled to are removed and examined for cancer. If they are cancer free, then the cancer is unlikely to have spread to the lymph nodes. [6]

Genetic Testing and Molecular Typing

You may have bloodwork performed to determine genetic markers you might carry that were inherited from your parents that could be implicated in cancer and be passed on to your children. This type of testing is also known as germline testing. One mutation that many people are familiar with is the mutations in the BRCA1 and BRCA2 genes that are implicated in a host of cancers including breast, ovarian, and pancreas. Mutations can make it more likely that you could get cancer but can also help to select treatments your cancer is more likely to respond to and can allow for your family members to be screened for these mutations. Next generation sequencing allows

While genetic mutations may increase your risk of cancer, some genetic mutations respond well to certain cancer treatments.

your DNA to be quickly evaluated to determine the types of therapies might be most effective to improve cancer outcomes.[7]

Genetic testing checks multiple genes that may be relevant in the treatment of cancer. Typically, a patient's personal history and family history is used by a genetic counselor to help to decide which genes should be studied. For example, because my mother's father also had pancreatic cancer, several genetic mutations that are implicated in pancreatic cancer were checked. The genetic counselor will meet with you prior to your testing, where he or she will explain to you what you are being tested for and what the significance of those genetic markers might be. Afterwards, you will sign the consent form to have the genetic testing. The genetic counselor will call you with the results of your genetic testing. If your genetic testing comes up positive for certain germline mutations, your first-degree relatives such as your parents, siblings, or children should also be tested for this mutation.

In addition to germline testing, it might be suggested that your tumor be molecularly typed. Molecular typing, also known as somatic testing, tests for genetic factors that might be embedded within the tumor itself.[8] These tumor mutations are not mutations that can be inherited. Molecular profiling assesses the genetic material of a tumor - its DNA and RNA as well as proteins. Molecular profiling can be performed on tissue from solid tumors taken

> **Even if you do not carry a genetic mutation in your DNA, your cancer can express a genetic mutation.**

during a biopsy or on tumor cells that are circulating in the blood.[8] I encourage you to insist on molecular typing so that your biopsy can be used to help guide your treatment.

Molecular profiling allows for personalized or precision medicine. One company doing molecular profiling is FoundationOne which can be found at the

website https://www.foundationmedicine.com/.
[9] This testing allows for more targeted therapy. For example, if a tumor is microsatellite unstable high, then that opens up potential treatments that will be more effective. Approximately 24 cancers at this point have microsatellite instability treatment options.[8] Always keep a copy of your report. Keep a copy even if your tumor does not show any mutations with current treatments. Keep a copy even if the molecular profiling finds mutations for which it is not understood whether it plays a role in cancer or treatment – these will be noted as VUS or variant of unknown significance. There might be a treatment that is developed later on that could help. For example, my mom did not carry mutations in the BRCA1/BRCA2 genes, but her tumor did. Two years after her diagnosis, a medication was approved for BRCA1 and BRCA2 tumors. Today, many cancer-specific support groups have tumor type registries where you can actually register your molecular profile.

CT Scan

A computerized tomagraphy (CT) scan takes pictures of slices or cross sections of your body.[10] A CT scan can show a tumor size, shape and location. CT scans are like x rays and uses an energy beam to create pictures from different angles. CT scans might be given with contrast (a form of color dye) to get a better picture of the tumor. Contrast might be swallowed, given by IV, or an enema.[10]

PET Scan

Positron emission tomography or PET scan is another type of diagnostic testing. PET scans may be used in place of CT scans. While a CT scans and an MRI show anatomical details including tumor size, PET scans show tumor activity.[11] Because of this, PET scans can help determine if a tumor is cancerous or not. Typically, a radioactive sugar (glucose) solution is ingested. Tumor cells tend to uptake glucose in greater amounts because they need sugar as fuel to help them divide. [11] It may be recommended that both a PET scan and a CT scan be performed in order to help to understand a tumor size as well as tumor activity.

Ports

Chemotherapy (chemo) may be given intravenously (IV).[12] While IV lines can be run through a vein in your body, they can also be placed in a port, or central venous catheter. Having a port placed helps you to have your cancer treatment without experiencing vein damage. A port is typically placed inside your chest into a large vein near your heart. There is an access area at the end of the port just under your skin where a nurse can insert a special needle to run the chemo medications through an intravenous (IV) line and can also draw blood from here. Your port can stay in for as long as you're getting treatment and even after as long as it is being flushed out once a month. Another, less common, way you can have your chemo administered is through a peripherally inserted central catheter (PICC line) which is inserted into your arm and into a vein which connects to a large vein near your heart. A PICC sticks out of your arm through your skin with the dressing covering it.[12]

Chemotherapy

The term chemo refers to any medication that is used to treat cancer. [13] Chemo has been in development since the early 1900s.[14] It was only in the 1960s where chemo was thought to be able to cure cancer and by the 1970s chemo was being used in conjunction with other treatments such as surgery and radiation. Chemo began to reduce cancer mortality, particularly in the final decades of the 20th century.[14]

Chemo can be infused via IV or can be given in the form of a pill, shot or cream. Chemo is a systemic treatment; the medications travel throughout the body. [13] While chemo can be used at any stage of cancer, it is the first line of defense in stage four cancer because the cancer is systemic and so is chemo. The goals of chemo could be used to cure a disease, to control a disease, or for alleviation of symptoms. Alleviation of symptoms is called palliative care. Chemotherapy can shrink a tumor prior to having radiation and can be used after surgery or radiation to kill any remaining cancer cells. [13]

While your goal with treatment is always to reach the status of NED, chemo can also be used if NED is not reached or if a cancer recurrence is experienced. [13] The type of chemo you have will be based on what type of cancer you have and if genetic testing revealed any mutations in your genes or the tumor that might respond to certain medications better. Other factors that will be taken into account are the stage of your cancer, your age, your overall health and medications you take, what other medical conditions you might have, and what other types of treatment you had for your cancer in the past. Your overall health will be assessed using the Eastern Cooperative Oncology Group (ECOG) Perfomance Status. (Table 3.2) Your oncologist, or cancer doctor, will balance the highest dosage that can be tolerated to kill cancer while still minimizing these side effects.[13]

Side effects from chemo range from mild to severe.[16] The duration of side effects can be short lived to taking months or years to resolve. Because chemo targets cancer cells which divide quickly, it also will target healthy cells that happen to divide quickly such as bone marrow cells that form blood, hair follicles, and cells in the mouth, digestive tract and reproductive system. As a result, chemo can cause hair loss, digestive issues like diarrhea and constipation and mouth sores. In addition to these side effects, other common side effects of chemo include fatigue, bruising, infections, nausea and vomiting, pain with swallowing, weight changes, concentration issues (sometimes called "chemo brain"), changes in fertility, and tingling or numbness in the hands and feet. More severe effects of chemo can include organ damage such as damage to the heart, kidneys, and lungs. There may be medication that can help to counteract these side effects as well.[16]

Metronomic chemo calculates a dose that will cause the maximum reduction of a tumor while minimizing the toxicity of chemo.[17] Metronomic chemo might be more effective than conventional chemo and may increase the tumor cells receptivity to the medication. This type of chemo works by periodically depriving the cancer cells from the chemo and prevents the cancer cells from adapting and surviving while chemo is being continuously administered. Metronomic chemo is administered frequently at a low dose over a long period of time. Another approach might start off on a very low dose and gradually increase the dosage during a chemotherapy treatment to reduce the tumor cells' resistance to the chemo drug.[17]

Table 3.2 ECOG Performance Status[15]

Grade	Performance Status
0	Fully active, able to carry on all pre-disease performance without restriction
1	Restricted in physically strenuous activity but ambulatory and able to carry out work of a light or sedentary nature (light housework, office work)
2	Ambulatory and capable of all selfcare but unable to carry out any work activities; up and about more than 50% of waking hours
3	Capable of only limited selfcare; confined to bed or chair more than 50% of waking hours
4	Completely disabled; cannot carry on any selfcare; totally confined to bed or chair

Radiation

Radiation therapy is one type of cancer treatment in which high-energy radiation is used to damage the DNA in cancer cells.[18] This damage prevents cancer cells from dividing and spreading. Radiation therapy affect the immune system of a cancer tumor, as the cell death caused by radiation is in part related to the immune system.[19] Radiation targets the tumor environment by activating the immune system and assisting in cell death.[19] Because of this immune system activation, radiation may be used with immunotherapy to increase the effectiveness of radiation. [19] Radiation is more targeted therapy. For this reason, if it is used in the case of stage 4 cancer, it is used for palliative purposes to alleviate symptoms such as pain. Because radiation is targeted, it preferentially damages cancer cells, that are not as good at repairing themselves like healthy cells.[18]

Sometimes radiation is used in combination with surgery, chemotherapy or even immunotherapy.[18] It can be used before surgery to shrink a tumor. It can be used after surgery to destroy any cancer cells that might remain. Radiation is commonly externally administered, although sometimes it can also be delivered inside the body through a catheter or through seeds that are implanted in the tumor, as in the cases of a gynecological or prostate cancer.[18]

Surgery

Surgery may be performed to remove your tumor or reduce the size of a tumor to either make treatments work better or to ease cancer symptoms.[20] Surgery might involve cutting out the tumor under local, regional or general anesthesia. Cryosurgery uses extremely cold gas to kill abnormal tumors or cells. Lasers can precisely cut out small areas of cancerous tissue on the skin or on the lining of your organs.[20] Surgery can be performed to remove an entire tumor to reduce the tumor.

Stem Cell Transplant

A stem cell transplant is sometimes called a bone marrow transplant. This procedure is used for blood disorders that include blood cancers such as leukemia. Stem cell transplants replace bone marrow after a high dose of chemo is used to destroy the cancerous bone marrow. Stem cell transplants can be autologous, in which your own stem cells or used, or allogenic in which donor stem cells are used. [21] Stem cells can also be obtained from umbilical cord blood. Stem cells can be harvested from bone marrow in the pelvis during a surgical procedure or from the blood, after injections that promote stem cell production in the bone marrow. [21]

Irreversible electroporation

Irreversible electroporation, or Nanoknife, is a method for killing localized tumors and can also be used for metastases to help to control the spread of disease.[22] This technique uses strong electrical fields to create microscopic pores in the cell membrane of tumors. These pores disrupt the stability of the cancer cells because the pores stay open, causing complete cell death. The advantage of irreversible electroporation is that it avoids damage to other tissues, such as organs and blood vessels and only damages the cancer cells being targeted. The treatment is minimally invasive and is typically performed with some sort of guidance via ultrasound, CT scan, or MRI. Ultrasound and CT scan can help with performing the procedure and CT scan, ultrasound, and MRI can be used to evaluate tumor tissue damage after the procedure. Irreversible electroporation is typically administered under general anesthesia because you need to remain completely still during the procedure. Common uses for this procedure include treating liver cancer as well as liver metastases, pancreatic cancer as well as tumors in the lung, kidney and GI tract. [22]

Hyperthermia

Hyperthermia exposes small areas of the body to high temperatures. This can kill cancer cells or damage them to make them more likely to respond to treatment. Radiofrequency ablation (RFA) is a type of hyperthermia which uses high energy radio waves to generate heat. Photodynamic therapy kills tumors by exposing them to light in combination with medications that react to that light.

Molecular Profile-specific Therapy

There are several types of treatment that can be provided based on the results of your genetic testing. Immunotherapy, cancer vaccines and gene therapy are all types of treatment that may be offered. Depending on the type of molecular-targeted therapy, it can interfere with specific molecules to prevent cancer growth, cell division, and metastases; interfere with cancer cell metabolism, induce cell death, or alter the environment of the actual cancer tumor through blocking the blood supply the tumor needs to grow.[26]

Immunotherapy

Immunotherapy is a cancer treatment that works together with your body's natural defenses - your immune system - to help you fight cancer.[24,25] The main focus of immunotherapy is to activate inactive immune cells that surround the cancer to help to destroy cancer cells.[25] Immune checkpoint inhibitor monoclonal antibody treatments can increase the production of your own antibodies or can act as antibodies themselves. These antibodies target and block the activity of abnormal protein and cancer cells.[24,25] One subset of monoclonal antibodies are antibody drug conjugates. These direct medication to cancer cells by binding an antibody to smaller anti-cancer drugs. This also can indirectly cause the body to recruit cells that break down the dead cancer cells, which in turn triggers the immune system to also attack cancer cells.[23] The antibodies will target and deliver the drugs directly to the cancer cells. Other targeted immunotherapy can even focus on cancer specific genes, or proteins, or even the environment that helps a tumor grow and survive.[25]

PARP inhibitors can work with monoclonal antibody therapy to increase its effectiveness.[26] PARP is an enzyme in cells that helps cells to repair damage. By blocking PARP through the use of a PARP inhibitor, cancer cells cannot repair any damage that cancer treatment induces.[25]

Nonspecific immunotherapies are also made in a lab can also help your immune system destroy cancer cells.[24] Nonspecific immunotherapy can use proteins to tell your body that there is a foreign invader and help your immune system destroy cancer cells and slow the growth of tumor. These therapies can help your cells talk to each other and mount an immune response.[24]

Oncolytic virus therapy changes viruses in a lab to destroy cancer cells.[24] The genetically modified virus is injected into the tumor. When the virus enters the cancer cells, it makes copies of itself, destroying cancer cells. The cancer cell death causes your own immune system to start to target any extra cancer cells in your body that have the same proteins as the cancer cells that were targeted.[24]

Car-T cell therapy is another type of immunotherapy.[24] The T cells in your body fight infection. In this type of therapy, your T cells are removed from your blood and proteins are added to your T cells in a lab. These proteins help the T cells to recognize cancer cells. When these T cells are injected back into your body, they help to find and destroy cancer cells.[24] There are also cancer vaccines out there that help your body fight disease[24] and cancer vaccines being tested in clinical trials.[23] Patient-specific cancer vaccines are made from the patient's own tumor cells. Non-specific vaccines create an immune response and may also have an anti-tumor effect.[23] Just like other vaccines, these cancer vaccines expose your immune system to a foreign protein which is called an antigen. This antigen triggers an antibody response in your immune system that helps your body find and destroy the cancer.[24]

Gene therapy

Gene therapy inserts either DNA or RNA into cancer cells. The DNA or RNA can work to destroy cancer cells or to reduce cancer cell division. Gene therapy can either replacing genes that have mutations with normal genes or introducing genetic material that can cause an immune system response.[23]

Clinical Trials

You may wish to participate in a clinical trial. Some people choose to participate in a clinical trial right away, particularly if their cancer is advanced and has poor treatment options. Others may wish to participate in a clinical trial in order to access more recent innovations in cancer treatment, or established cancer treatments being used in new combinations. Clinical trials range from exploratory trials to advanced trials. There are typically four phases of a clinical trial that are open to human participation.[27] Phase 0 is exploring if and how a new drug works in order to speed up the approval process. Phase 0 trials only need to give a few doses to a few people; this phase is not widely used. Phase 1 clinical trials determine treatment safety by seeing if severe side effects occur and to observe what the drug does to the body. Phase 2 clinical trials examine treatment effectiveness. If a drug makes it through a phase 1 clinical trial, a phase 2 trial determines if a drug can cause cancer to shrink, disappear, or stabilize cancer growth. Phase 2 clinical trials typically enroll 25 to 100 patients. Everyone in a phase 2 trial will get the investigational drug. Phase 3 clinical trials study if the new treatment is better than what is already the standard of care. These trials are typically run as randomized clinical trials in which you either will receive the standard treatment or a new treatment. Phase 3 clinical trials enroll several hundred people and typically are run at multiple sites. Unlike phase 1 and 2 trials, phase 3 clinical trials are more likely to be widely offered in community hospitals and doctors' offices. A placebo medication is never used by itself in a phase 3 trial, so everyone enrolled will receive some type of cancer treatment. When a placebo is used, it would be used in conjunction with a standard chemo medication. This typically occurs if a new drug is being investigated for efficacy when paired with an established chemo regimen. If the results of a phase 3 clinical trial indicate that the new treatment has better results than the standard of care, then a new drug application is submitted. Phase 4 clinical trials are cleared by the Food and Drug Administration (FDA) and are watched over a long period of time. These trials study the long-term effects of a drug and typically enroll several thousand people. Patients can access medications that are used in phase 4 trial without being in a study, you would get the same care regardless of participation. The care you would get in a phase 4 clinical trials is the same as if you were to get treatment outside of the trial.[27] Most insurance plans cover the cost of approved clinical trials if you are eligible. Insurance plans differ on out of network coverage, so you should check with your insurance company if a clinical trial involves doctors or hospitals not in your network.

Your oncologist might call your attention to a clinical trial, particularly if they are associated with an academic medical center. I believe that it is also in your interest to periodically search for clinical trials. My mom's oncologist was a good oncologist, but he was also very busy and while he would periodically look to see if clinical trials were available for my mom, he was not necessarily up to date on the trials at any given moment. He was, after all, a clinician and not a researcher. Another important point about clinical trials is that while you might not want to enroll in a Phase 1 or 2 trial because the safety or effectiveness of a treatment isn't yet established. Seeing what phase 1 and 2 trials are running might give you a better picture of future phase 3 trials in which you might want to participate.

The FDA has a program for expanded access or compassionate access for investigational drugs which allows for patients with advanced cancer to access drugs that are currently in clinical trials.[28] Compassionate use of medication requires the review and permission by the FDA and cooperation of both the drug manufacturer and the patient's health care providers. The FDA employs people whose sole job is to work with patients and their doctors to permit the access to compassionate use drugs.[28]

There are several resources that you can use to search for clinical trials that might be right for you. The Center for Information and Study of Clinical Research Participation has a free "Find a Trial" feature located at this

webpage
https://www.ciscrp.org/services/search-clinical-trials/search-trials-now/.[29] The National Cancer Institute has a website that can help you find National Cancer Institute supported clinical trials. It has a search engine that allows you to type in the type of cancer you have, can type in your age, and your zip code.[30] This search engine can be found at https://www.cancer.gov/about-cancer/treatment/clinical-trials/search.[30] Clinical trials.gov is another database of both privately and publicly funded international clinical trials.[31] You can set restrictions on the country, can search by disease, and can even search by a clinical trial number, name, or investigator name.

Cancer-specific groups can be useful for helping you find clinical trials for your specific cancer as well. For example, we used the Pancreatic Cancer Action Network (PanCan) to run a clinical trial search for us shortly after diagnosis and a year and a half after diagnosis.[32] This saved a lot of time because their service took down information such as how far we were willing to travel, cancer stage, and types of treatments my mom had already had in order to find trials that were enrolling and for which my mom met the narrow criteria.

Some oncologists might be more abreast of current clinical trials and others may not be. If your oncologist is not up to date on the most recent clinical trials, it might just demonstrate that they are a very busy treating cancer with the best-known, available treatment. Your oncologist is a clinician and may not be involved in research; clinicians spend their day giving their patients the best care available for their particular cancer and stage. Because of this, you should not solely rely on your oncologist for information about clinical trials. Coming into your appointments armed with trials and their inclusion and exclusion criteria - the criteria of who can and cannot participate in a trial - will help you and your oncologist have a discussion as to which options might be good for your now or later on in your treatment.

No matter what your cancer stage, you should understand the rationale behind the treatments being offered. Your oncologist should provide you with a list of the options and discuss how each one works, what they recommend, and why. You might want to do your own research on PubMed.gov to better understand standard treatments and results of clinical trials for your type of cancer prior to your appointment.[33] If your practitioner does not respect you for taking a decision-making role in the partnership, you might want to evaluate if that partnership is the right one for your care. The oncologist might be the expert in cancer in your partnership, but you are the owner and operator of your body. You should identify your own goals for your health and happiness and select a treatment that aligns with these goals.[34]

While the stage of your cancer will somewhat dictate what type of treatment is appropriate, you will still have options at each stage. When considering choosing a cancer treatment, you should consider what the end point or desired outcome of your cancer treatment is. Will your cancer treatment allow you to have better quality of life? Will it allow you to live longer? Living longer without a high quality of life might not necessarily be a goal. When selecting a treatment or considering participation in a clinical trial, you should consider having improvements in both your survival and your quality of life. Other endpoints that are things to consider when choosing a treatment option are progression-free survival, where your cancer is not cured but is also not growing or spreading or disease-free survival in which you achieve NED and live for a while with that status.

❖ ❖ ❖ ❖ ❖ ❖ ❖ ❖ ❖ ❖ ❖ ❖ ❖ ❖ ❖ ❖ ❖ ❖
Notes and Questions
❖ ❖ ❖ ❖ ❖ ❖ ❖ ❖ ❖ ❖ ❖ ❖ ❖ ❖ ❖ ❖ ❖ ❖

Chapter 4 Assembling Your Healthcare Team

Your healthcare team needs to provide you with the correct type of support. The members of your healthcare team should listen to your concerns and treat you as a whole human being and not as just another cancer to be treated.[1] Your oncologist should listen to your concerns; provide you with information; and partner with you to make the healthcare decisions that best align with your goals.[1] Your healthcare team should provide you with all of the information about your diagnosis and treatment so that you can make appropriate decisions and know what to expect from those treatment decisions. They should not abruptly withdraw support once your cancer is successfully treated, as this can cause anxiety.[1]

In our own search for providers, my mom assembled a healthcare team that aligned with her goal to have good quality of life; to prolong her life; and to attempt to slow or stop the growth of her cancer. She wanted to remain active and participate in her activities; continue helping homeschool my daughters; and go to brunches and dinners with friends. Her healthcare team consisted of her oncologist, an acupuncturist, a hypnotherapist trained in cognitive behavioral therapy, an integrative physician who treated patients with cancer, and a physician that gave her high-dose, IV vitamin

C. My mom also had access to my expertise as a physical therapist. We had some other great holistic consults with whom we did not pursue treatment for very long, as my mom's intuition was that it was not the right path for her to take.[2] This chapter covers a more traditional healthcare team. An in-depth treatment of holistic providers will occur in Chapter 6.

Oncologist

You will have an oncologist as part of your medical team. An oncologist is a type of doctor that specializes in cancer.[3] A medical oncologist deals with medications such as chemo or immunotherapy that treat your cancer. A radiation oncologist is the doctor that administers radiation therapy to treat your cancer. A surgical oncologist is the doctor that surgically removes tumors.[3]

Occupational Therapist

Occupational therapy can help you perform daily tasks, called activities of daily living, more easily.[4] These tasks are things like dressing, bathing and cooking. They can assess your skills and give you exercises to help you get stronger at these activities. They can recommend adaptive equipment and teach you how to use it to help you with your daily tasks.[4]

Oncology Social Worker

A licensed oncology social worker can help you manage day-to-day concerns such as meals or transportation to your care.[5] They can help you find grants to pay for your medicine and can help you fill out the forms so that you can receive Social Security disability payments. Oncology social workers can help support you emotionally through counseling or by finding you a support group.[5]

Physical Therapist

Physical therapists are movement experts who can provide appropriate exercise prescription to address cancer-related fatigue and improve your strength and mobility. Some physical therapists specialize in working with patients with cancer, while others work with a general population of people that includes patients with cancer.[6] Finding a physical therapist to help improve your overall physical activity level and function is an important step to your healing. If you live in the United States, you can use the "Find a PT" function at https://www.choosept.com/resources/choose.aspx. You can even select oncology as a specialty area to see if there is a nearby physical therapist who specializes in oncology. Chapter 7 discusses the importance of exercise in detail.

Psychologist

It is important to maintain hope even in the face of terminal disease. The language of cancer often involves "beating cancer" or "fighting cancer," which might not be helpful if you have elected hospice services and just want to feel at peace with your decision. Seeing a psychologist one-on-one or going to group therapy may alleviate stress and reinforce resilience. Cognitive Behavioral Therapy (CBT) can help you with problematic patterns of thinking so that you can reframe your viewpoint.[7,8] CBT can improve mood, fatigue, quality of life and cognition and reduce insomnia, anxiety and depression.[8,9] When paired with exercise, CBT can decrease cancer-related fatigue.[10] Another type of therapy called Acceptance and Commitment Therapy, or ACT, works to help a patient become comfortable with having thoughts or feelings that are challenging. ACT can help to reduce distress and improve mood and quality of life.[11]

Registered Dietician Nutritionist

An oncology registered dietician nutritionist will help you make better food choices. This will allow you take in enough calories with the best nutrients to keep you strong and feeling good.[12] They can answer your questions about food that will give you the best benefit in terms of staying strong, maintaining your weight, and taking in the right types of nutrients to help you during and after cancer treatment. They can decide if you need supplements such as vitamins or premade drinks to help support your nutrition.[12] You can find a registered dietician nutritionist near you at the following website https://www.eatright.org/find-an-expert.[13]

Respiratory Therapist

Respiratory therapists diagnose and recommend treatment for breathing disorders.[14] They can check out the oxygen levels found in blood and exhaled breath to determine treatment effectiveness and the need for a change in treatment plan. Respiratory therapists may work with patients with lung cancer and may also help screen for lung cancer.

Speech-Language Pathologist

A speech language pathologist can help you if you have difficulty or are unable to communicate due to your cancer or cancer treatment.[15] They can also help diagnose and treat swallowing disorders that might result from treatments such as surgery or radiation to the head or neck.

Hospice v. Palliative Care

Many people get confused about the terms hospice and palliative care and think they mean the same thing. My mom was confused on this point constantly and left our first appointment extremely upset that the first oncologist was offering her hospice. In actuality, she was offered her palliative chemotherapy to try to shrink her tumor and give her a longer life despite having stage IV cancer. Hospice is typically given when curative treatment is no longer possible. Hospice can help make the last months of life more comfortable with high quality of life.[16] To be placed on hospice, your oncologist will certify that you have 6 months or less to live; this is just an estimate and if you exceed that 6-month prediction you can still receive hospice services. Palliative care, or comfort care, includes patients at any stage of disease and is used to manage symptoms of chronic diseases, including cancer. Patients

Palliative care is not the same as hospice care. Palliative care manages the symptoms of chronic diseases, including cancer.

receiving palliative care can still pursue curative treatment. Palliative care is a part of hospice care in that it is managing symptoms to allow for better quality of life. Starting palliative care early in your treatment has a greater benefit than only using palliative care if you need hospice. [16] The National Hospice and Palliative Care Organization can be a valuable resource to finding both types of services and can be accessed at https://www.nhpco.org/patients-and-caregivers/.[17]

❖❖❖❖❖❖❖❖❖❖❖❖❖❖❖❖❖❖❖
Notes and Questions
❖❖❖❖❖❖❖❖❖❖❖❖❖❖❖❖❖❖❖

Chapter 5 Second and Third Opinions

My mom and I were committed to the idea of getting at least a second opinion even before the first opinion had disregarded my mom's goals. It was important to the both of us that her treatment be confirmed by a second set of eyes. Her second opinion oncologist was who we stayed with because he listened to what she wanted. He also wanted to be certain that mom truly had pancreatic cancer versus a benign cyst or a metastasis to her pancreas. The third opinion oncologist provided some information about how mom was microsatellite unstable-low and how that somewhat reduced her treatment options. This was helpful information as I could disregard clinical trials with high instability as the criteria. Each of these opinions provided us with a little more information to make our initial course of treatment clear.

You might worry about how the first oncologist would feel about your seeking a second opinion. The majority of patients seek a second opinion and at least half of patients seek a second opinion to confirm the initial

> **The majority of patients seek a second opinion. You owe it to yourself to make sure you feel confident in your diagnosis and treatment choices.**

opinion.[1] Patients want to be involved in making informed decisions using that shared decision-making model discussed in chapter 3 and oncologists have come to expect that you would seek a second opinion. One study found that 75% of physicians reacted favorably to the news that their patient was seeking a second opinion.[1] Other benefits of a second opinion are feelings of assurance in the plan of care and enhanced trust of the first physician.[1] Patients who feel that their oncologist respects their autonomy have higher satisfaction with their oncologist.[2] Improved satisfaction can lead to better quality of life, which in turn positively influences health. You owe it to yourself to make sure you feel confident in your diagnosis and treatment choices. There are some patients who may avoid a second opinion because they may trust the first physician they consult with or may not understand the purpose of a second opinion.[1]

With the internet, there is no limit to the amount of information patients have at their fingertips. While a large majority may receive information about their cancer from their oncologists, a good portion of patients find information in print media and the internet.[1] It is important to make sure that your information is coming from reliable health sources on the internet such as the websites listed in this book. For example, the results of clinical trials are frequently published in PubMed as are clinical trial protocols, so PubMed may be an important source of information for you on treatments in development.

Patients may be more likely to discuss cancer decisions with their friends and family before talking to their oncologist about their decisions. Family and friends might be encouraging you to seek a second opinion to make sure you have all of the information you need to make the best decision.[3] Patients may feel confident and satisfied with the information they receive from their oncologist about their planned treatment but may feel uncertain about the reason they have cancer, which may impede their overall satisfaction. A desire for better communication is commonly cited as the driving force behind a second opinion.[4] One study found that less than half of all patients were satisfied with all aspects of information other than their planned treatment.[1] Communication is so important that patients will often choose the physician who they perceive as a better communicator, even in the case of identical diagnosis and treatment plans.[4] Many perceive that their second opinion was longer and that more of their questions were answered.[5] This was certainly the case with my mom's second opinion. The surgical oncologist spent a half hour with us, the oncology nurse spent significant time with us and the next day the medical oncologist spent a half hour with us. If you feel that you are missing information, bring a list of questions to your appointment and make sure your oncologist answers them. If your oncologist does not have time to answer your questions, this may indicate that you will not have a shared decision-making relationship. Some questions that you might consider asking at your second opinion can be found in box 5.1

Box 5.1 Questions for a Second Opinion Appointment

Based on the information in my medical file, do you agree with the original opinion?

What is your opinion of my prognosis?

Do you recommend any additional blood work?

Do you recommend any additional imaging?

What treatment would you recommend and why?

Are you aware of any clinical trials that would be appropriate for me?

My mom's question was always "If I was your mother, what would you recommend?" You could substitute father, sister, or brother for mother.

There are many reasons that you might have for wanting a second opinion. Typical positive motivations cited for a second opinion include a need for reassurance about a diagnosis, a desire to verify a proposed treatment plan, a need for personalized information including prognosis, and a desire to be seen by the best physician.[3-6] Patients want access to treatment options and information about the cancer diagnosis itself. A second opinion gives patients information about clinical trials and to have their information entered in a different hospital system for potential clinical trials. Other motivations include a lack of trust in their initial physician, dissatisfaction in communication, and a lack of a clear direction for treatment after their first opinion.[3,6] These second opinions help patients be better prepared to make an informed decision.

One consideration is that many hospitals have interdisciplinary tumor boards that evaluate cancer cases. These boards are comprised of various oncologists, pathologists, and radiologists who exchange information about each patient case that is brought before them and sometimes serve as a second opinion for some patients.[7] Because many hospitals not affiliated with the National Cancer Institute do not have tumor boards, you should ask if a tumor board will be reviewing your case. While a second opinion will typically confirm your original diagnosis and treatment plan, on some occasions it may change your diagnosis or course of treatment. One study examined the charts of 70 women with breast

Ask your oncologist if a tumor board will be reviewing your case

cancer seeking second opinions, in which less than 10% had their first opinion from an academic medical setting. Over half of the women seeking second opinions had additional imaging or biopsy recommendations made, approximately 15% of patients were referred for genetic testing, 23% had an additional cancer found, and 20% of patients had a change in pathology interpretation. The diagnosis was revised in 43% of the patients seeking second opinions.[7] Another study looking at second opinions in endometrial cancer found small differences in diagnoses, tumor type, and staging which changed clinical management in some cases.[8] A study in the Netherlands found the majority of second opinions were initiated by patients and that those patients had not undergone treatment before getting a second opinion.[9] This study also found a little less than half of patients had a discrepancy in opinion. While the majority of discrepancies were in tumor staging, about 30% of these discrepancies were due to differences in the proposed treatment. Most patients in this study stayed with the second opinion oncologist, which may be because the second opinion hospital was a cancer research institution with a high level of expertise.[9] This highlights that seeking an opinion at a cancer research institution may provide greater confidence in the course of care. It should be noted that there is a wide range of 2-51% of reported discrepancies in opinions noted in the medical literature.[6,10]

The reality in seeking opinions and medical care is that not everyone has the same financial resources. This can impact whether you can travel to seek second opinions or if you can afford to complement your traditional cancer treatment with holistic therapies. Limited financial resources can influence differences in both the type of care offered and second opinion seeking. For example, one study found that patients with esophageal cancer who had lower socioeconomic status were less likely to be offered surgery and were less likely to seek a second opinion.[11] Lower educational level is also associated with decreased rates of second opinion seeking [1,3] An additional challenge that patients of less financial means faced was that they were more likely to lose their jobs, placing a financial strain through loss of income and loss of medical

Ask your oncologist if there is a financial counselor or case management social worker available to provide guidance regarding your medical bills.

insurance. However, when patients are offered a case management social worker they are able to resolve their financial issues that impacted cancer care.[11] Regardless of your income or insurance status, you should ask your oncologist if there is a financial counselor or case management social worker available to provide guidance regarding your medical bills.

Getting a second opinion, even if you stay with your first oncologist and your treatment and diagnosis does not change, can be a valuable tool to gain a deeper understanding of your disease.[12] A second opinion allows you to become more active in making decisions about your cancer. Second opinions also help other patients, as the more patients who oncologists see, the better understanding they have of cancer, including patients whose response to treatment is better than expected or unusual in some way. [12]

Your desire for more information about your diagnosis and choices is normal and can help you receive better health care.[4] Getting a second opinion will help you get more involved in the decision-making process and resolve self-doubt and fear [4,10] The book Radical Remission talks about taking control of your health. It reinforces the idea that you need to be willing to make changes in your life and make decisions in partnership rather than in response to your oncologist.[10] Taking an active versus a passive role in your health will lead to more positive health outcomes for you and promote healing. [10]

❖❖❖❖❖❖❖❖❖❖❖❖❖❖❖❖❖❖❖
Notes and Questions
❖❖❖❖❖❖❖❖❖❖❖❖❖❖❖❖❖❖❖

Chapter 6 Holistic Treatments

The benefits of homeopathy on health and wellbeing, including cancer care, are well described.[1] The term complementary and alternative medicine (CAM) describes a wide range of treatment modalities that is outside of

> Complementary and Alternative Medicine encompasses a wide range of treatments outside the realm of conventional Western medicine

the realm of conventional Western medicine. [2] CAM can be used in conjunction with or instead of traditional Western medicine treatments. The term integrative medicine is often used to describe the combination of treatments using both CAM and Western medicine; the use of integrative medicine is increasing in patients with cancer.[2] Most patients report doing some form of complementary treatment during the course of their cancer care.[1,3] One study found that over half of patients used CAM therapies at some point after their cancer diagnosis and a little less than half during their treatment.[4] Another study examined the use of integrative and complementary medicine in patients with breast and gynecological cancers and found that a little over half used these practices for general health and 41% used this to help treat their cancer.[5] The most commonly used treatments were supplements, homeopathic remedies, vitamins, and selenium. Patients most frequently want to see CAM, relaxation therapy, and dietary counseling offered along with their traditional cancer care.[5] Patients with cancer might use CAM to reduce side effects and promote their emotional well-being or may even use it to treat the cancer itself.[2,6] Clinical studies of homeopathic remedies combined with conventional care has shown that the remedies improve quality of life, reduce symptom burden, and possibly improve survival in patients with cancer.[7] There are many forms of holistic treatments. This chapter will go over some common types that patients living with cancer may choose and will give you resources to pursue the range of holistic treatments.

Integrative care should be introduced early on as part of cancer treatment. As discussed in Chapter 4, palliative care is not exclusive to hospice care, and is most effective at reducing side effects from cancer and cancer treatment when begun early after diagnosis. One study found the majority of patients seen in an integrative oncology service had significant improvement during cancer treatment with the use of homeopathy and integrative care.[1] Improvements were noted for hot flashes, nausea, depression, fatigue, and severe anxiety. Homeopathy has a very low incidence of side effects.[1] You may have to request referrals to CAM in your hospital system or seek these treatments independent of your oncologist. One pilot study examined the benefits of traditional oncology in combination with psycho-oncology and integrative medicine.[8] Over two-thirds of the patients in this study had distress that was at or exceeded the threshold for treatment, which would indicate that traditional oncology was not sufficient in addressing the emotional needs of patients.[8] The majority of patients in this study did not use CAM. The primary reason cited was because CAM was not offered to them, highlighting that patients may not even be aware that CAM could help to alleviate emotional distress, pain and side effects from cancer and cancer treatments.[8]

When you are choosing an oncologist, be sure to ask how open they are to complementary therapies. Even if you have no intention at that point of using holistic treatments, you should keep all of your options

> Ask your oncologist how open they are to complementary therapies. Keep all treatment options on the table.

on the table. The difference in philosophy between typical allopathic medicine, and integrative or holistic practitioners, could mean that complementary therapies are not discussed with you during the course of your oncologist visit. One study examined conventional medicine and complementary care practitioners' attitudes and knowledge about treatment risks.[9] The majority of both types of practitioners, including those with dual training, were aware of the adverse effects of complementary modalities. Most doctors and nurses thought it was too risky to combine complementary treatments with traditional cancer care, whereas a little over half with dual training and less than half of complementary care practitioners thought this. The majority of doctors and nurses neither encouraged nor discouraged the use of complementary treatment, and most conventional medicine practitioners were concerned about the safety profile of complementary treatments.[9] In contrast, only 1% of complementary practitioners would have discouraged the use of traditional treatments like chemo. [9] Oncology practitioners typically make treatment recommendations based on clinical practice guidelines and evidence-based literature for conventional treatment but may not seek out evidence for complementary cancer modalities.[10] This may add to the perception that there is no evidence for complementary treatment.

Healthcare professionals should ask their patients about all of the treatments they are pursuing including CAM and ask specifically about supplements, herbs, and vitamins. One study found that the majority of patients reported their oncologist didn't ask whether they were currently using CAM and didn't offer CAM as a treatment modality.[4] A little over half of patients spontaneously mentioned the use of complementary medicine to their oncologist, which means that a sizable number of patients had oncologists who were unaware of their patients' other treatments.[4] If your oncologist does not mention; is dismissive of; or is against this type of treatment altogether, you may be less honest about the treatment you are pursuing. Oncologists may worry about the quality of supplements, the potential interaction with cancer therapies, or perceive there is a lack of scientific evidence for these treatments.[9] Additionally, oncologists may not be familiar with the range of CAM therapies that have evidence for them.[9] You want to have effective communication with your oncologist; if you are reluctant to inform your oncologist about the holistic treatments you are pursuing, then this oncologist might not be the best fit. If you desire to stay with an oncologist who is skeptical of more holistic treatments, seeking out an integrative physician may alleviate these challenges, as an integrative physician that specializes in cancer care would be aware of potential interactions between conventional cancer treatment and homeopathic therapies. My mom's oncologist did not always agree with her holistic choices, but he was open to her use of the treatments.

Healthcare providers with a collaborative style allow for adequate information exchange, which can help a patient make informed decisions about

CAM/integrative care usage.[11] Communication styles affect patient satisfaction and distress, decision-making, well-being, and likelihood of following through with treatment recommendations and instructions.[11] CAM practitioners are often rated higher than physicians in aspects of listening and providing emotional support, which highlights that patients have needs that go beyond physical into the areas of social, emotional, financial and employment, and spiritual needs.[11]

CAM providers may ask you what conventional treatments have tried, which ones were successful and which ones were not, as well as about treatments you rejected based on factors such as how well they would impact your prognosis.[11] CAM practitioners may ask you about your spiritual or religious values and beliefs, what types of support you need on a consistent basis, and who is in your social network including family, friends, and community.[11] Ideally, your oncologist also will ask this second set of questions to better understand who you are.

You may feel overwhelmed about the range of holistic choices available to you. You may have concerns about

> A Moss Report discusses the scientific evidence for conventional cancer care and holistic treatments.

whether a holistic treatment is safe or effective. Additionally, many times complementary therapies are not covered by insurance, which may make it challenging to afford a range of treatments. This is where purchasing a Moss Report for your specific type of cancer may be useful (https://www.mossreports.com/). As of this writing a downloadable Moss Report was $389. These reports will discuss the scientific evidence for both conventional cancer care as well as various holistic treatments including infusions and supplements. The reports rate each treatment as red light where the treatment is dangerous, yellow light where there is some concern or where enough evidence isn't available, and green light in which safety and efficacy of the treatment has been demonstrated.[12] This may help you decide which holistic treatments to pursue, will give you safety ratings and references to discuss with your oncologist, and will increase your understanding of the various treatments out there so that you could discuss them with an integrative or naturopathic doctor.

Integrative Physician

Your first stop may be seeing an integrative physician. Integrative medicine focuses not on pathology impacting the physical body,[3] but rather identifies and addresses illness from a physical and energetic imbalance. The cause of the imbalance and the context from which this imbalance arose are examined in integrative medicine. Cancer would be viewed as a body in a system of imbalance due to internal or external causes. From this perspective, spirituality, diet, sleep, exercise, environmental exposures and toxins all can impact balance.[3]

Your integrative physician may either be a general practitioner or one who focuses on oncology. Integrative oncology is the practice of using both CAM and mainstream cancer treatments both during active cancer and into survivorship. This includes the use of nutrition, dietary and herbal supplements, acupuncture and Mind Body practices.[3] Research indicates that integrative oncology can play an important role in cancer treatment and can even improve survival.[1]. An integrative physician has expertise and training in treating the patient in view of their lifestyle and habits, rather than just treating a disease. Integrative physicians typically provide guidance not just on medications, but also on improving nutrition and supplements to promote health.[1] Integrative physicians may also direct you to other types of complementary medicine such as acupuncture or meditation.

If you consult with an integrative doctor, the doctor will ask questions to better understand your medical history. The doctor will also talk to you about what your expectations are with respect to integrative care. The doctor will ask about your cancer care to date and will give you time to ask questions and talk about any concerns you might have.[1]

Naturopathic doctor

Naturopathic doctors (NDs) are trained at a naturopathic medical school in diagnosis, prevention, and treatment of illness through supporting their patients' own ability to heal.[13] The tenets of naturopathy are to remove any obstacles to optimal health, stimulate the patient's ability to heal, strengthen the body systems that are weak, improve or maintain musculoskeletal integrity, restore health through natural substances, use medication to halt disease progression, and use invasive treatments to preserve life or function. Only 22 states license naturopathic doctors, which means that depending on the state you live in the ND may be able to prescribe medication or may need to refer you back to your medical doctor. Additionally, if the ND feels you need invasive treatment, they will refer you to your medical doctor. NDs may use a variety of treatments including botanical medicine, vitamins and supplements, nutrition, massage and manipulation, and holistic medicine to support the body's ability to heal itself.[13]

One study looked at NDs role in cancer care.[14] Common natural health products that were recommended included fish-derived omega-3 fatty acids, vitamin D, probiotics, melatonin, vitamin C, homeopathy, arnica, and tumeric/curcumin. Typical nutritional recommendations were anti-inflammatory diets, dairy restriction, Mediterranean diet, gluten restriction and ketogenic diet. Typical physical modalities recommended were exercise, acupuncture, acupressure, cranial sacral therapy, and yoga. Typical interventions to target mental health were meditation, art therapy, mindfulness-based stress reduction, music therapy and visualization therapy.[14]. You can use the American Association of Naturopathic Physician's Find a Doctor page (https://naturopathic.org/search/custom.asp?id=5613) if you are interested in exploring the role an ND may have in your cancer care.[15]

Care Oncology Clinic

The Care Oncology Clinic (COC) was started in London. There is now a US-based COC that serves patients in the United States and Canada. The COC protocol uses medications off-label to block the sugar, fat, and protein pathways that cancer uses to replicate. Off-label means the medication is being used for a purpose other than the intended use cleared by the FDA. These medications also promote better immune system functioning, block cancer cells' ability to repair damage, alters the ability of cancer cells to grow and divide, and induces cell death. I first learned of COC while reading Jane McClelland's book How to Starve Cancer: Without Starving Yourself, which I highly recommend.[16] McClelland is a UK-based physiotherapist who was diagnosed many years ago with Stage IV cancer. She developed a map for the use of off-label medications and supplements to essentially starve cancer cells and induce cancer cell death. She also advocates for exercise and improved nutrition. Her protocol is similar to that of the COC, which only uses off-label medications such as statins, metformin, and menbendazole, but does not use supplements. After reading this book, I was convinced that I needed to take my mom to London to be seen by COC and was happy to find out about the US-based clinic. We scheduled a consultation using their website https://careoncology.com/products/initial-consult-pre-pay/. [17] The consultation occurred via telehealth and then a doctor with prescribing capabilities in all 50 states wrote prescriptions for the off-label medications, which are common medications with few side effects. My mom was unable to stay with the protocol-the one medication Metformin, which is a medication used with Type 2 diabetes gave her gastrointestinal upset (a common side effect), even with the extended-release formula. My mom's pancreatic cancer was likely causing this intolerance. Had we found out about this protocol earlier, perhaps my mom would have tolerated it better. We tried substituting Metformin with a different supplement, but even that was not tolerable. Other barriers to using COC are the cost of the consultation and the cost of the medications, which are not covered by insurance due to their off-label usage. As of this writing the costs in US dollars were $800 for the initial consultation, followed by $295 for follow-up, and bundled medication costs of about $60.[18] The cost of the first year is $2390, with the following years being less expensive at $1880.[18] If you have a flexible spending account or healthcare savings account you may be able to be reimbursed for these costs. Advantages to this protocol are the attention that the consulting physician and oncology nurse support; the fact that it uses medications that have been in use for a long time and have few side effects; and the fact that you can continue this protocol while using conventional cancer care.

Focused Ultrasound Foundation

While ultrasound is a mainstream medical treatment, both for diagnosis as well as by physical and occupational therapists for treating musculoskeletal injuries, the application of ultrasound by the Focused Ultrasound Foundation is novel and thus I have included it in this chapter. The Focused Ultrasound Foundation uses ultrasound waves to accurately target tumors. Depending on the frequency of the waves used, anti-cancer effects include increasing an immune response, improving sensitivity of a tumor to chemotherapy, or even inducing cancer cell death.[19] This non-invasive treatment is paired with an MRI to provide doctors with a precise image of where the ultrasound should be focused. As of this writing, focused ultrasound is only approved by the FDA for the treatment of bone metastases; however, there are clinical trials for a wide range of cancers both in the United States and worldwide.[19] You can find a treatment site and clinical trials through their treatment sites search page https://www.fusfoundation.org/the-technology/treatment-sites.[20]

Berkson Protocol

While this chapter will not have an extensive list of supplements for cancer care, there will be a few that I highlight. The first is the Berkson protocol, which utilizes supplements, IV vitamin C and alpha lipoic acid (ALA), and low dose naltrexone.[21-24] ALA dosages ranging from 300 to 600 mg is given by IV. [21] ALA is contained in many enzymes and is involved in cell metabolism, can reduce oxidative stress, can inhibit cancer cell growth, and can induce cancer cell death. ALA also promotes immune cell function.[22] Low dose naltrexone (LDN) in doses of 3.0 to 4.5 mg is taken before bedtime blocks the body's opiate receptors for a brief time, during which the body produces large amounts of opiates to stimulate the cells of the immune system, and may slow tumor growth and stabilize disease.[22,23] I should note that because LDN blocks opioid receptors, if you are in need of opioid pain medication for your cancer, you cannot also take LDN. This highlights why communication with all of your doctors is so important. High dose vitamin C is given via IV; vitamin C in low doses is an antioxidant that reduces inflammation, but in high doses also produces hydrogen peroxide, which causes oxidative stress that can kill cancer cells. High dose vitamin C is more readily absorbed if given in an IV. IV vitamin C may increase overall survival and progression-free survival.[25] The Berkson protocol also prescribes daily oral antioxidant supplements of 600 mg of ALA daily, 200 mcg of selenium twice daily and silymarin 300 mg 4 times a day.[22]

I tried to get my mom into the Berkson clinic in New Mexico, but they were only seeing in-state patients due to the commitment of travel periodically. Fortunately, we were able to find people willing to do the infusions in our home state-two of the providers accessed my mom's port for the IV infusions. My mom took LDN throughout her cancer, did ALA and Vitamin C in the beginning and end of her cancer care and just high dose vitamin C treatments every week or every other week for about a year and a half in the middle. She really felt like these were the treatments that improved her survival and well-being.

Supplements

There are many supplements other than the ones in the Berkson protocol that have evidence for being beneficial in cancer care. I will talk about a few in this section that we found beneficial; however, understand that the list of all of the potential supplements useful in cancer care is quite extensive and beyond the scope of this book. I recommend that you talk to an integrative

> There are many potential supplements that can be beneficial for people who have cancer. Talk to an integrative physician or naturopathic doctor who can prescribe the right supplements for your particular cancer

physician or naturopathic doctor who can prescribe supplements that might be vitamins, botanical extracts, or other herbal remedies specific to your type of cancer.[26] A Moss Report will also help provide some guidance.[12]

Cannabinoids can help to reduce cancer pain and nausea and improve appetite.[3] The human body produces its own cannabinoids; however, cannabinoids can be introduced though certain types of mushrooms and fungi, ecchinacea, hemp (CBD) or marijuana (THC). Each state has its own regulations regarding the use of marijuana for medicinal purposes and may require that you have a doctor's prescription to access this treatment.[3] CBD on its own may reduce inflammation and CBD plus THC may play a role in limiting cancer growth and promoting cancer cell death as well as the clean-up of damaged cancer cells.[27,28]

Vitamin D has many anticancer properties and plays an important role in immune system function.[29] Vitamin D can be obtained from exposure to sunlight; foods like fish, egg yolks, and mushrooms; fortified foods such as orange juice, milk, tofu and cereal; and by taking a supplement.[30] Adequate Vitamin D levels are associated with decreased risk of cancer.[31] Evidence suggests that Vitamin D can prevent tumor initiation and growth through antioxidant, anti-inflammatory, and DNA-repair pathways.[29] Additionally, Vitamin D promotes cancer cell death and the clearing of damaged cells.[29] Vitamin D may improve survival after a cancer diagnosis and supplementation with Vitamin D may help to reduce mortality. [30,31] One study that combined the results of 50 trials found a 15% reduced risk of death from cancer.[32] While not all studies supported the use of vitamin D supplementation as solely able to reduce cancer risk and mortality,[33] researchers suggest that taking 2000 iu/day of Vitamin D may play a role in survival.[34]

Melatonin helps regulate your circadian rhythm or sleep-wake cycle.[35] The main place melatonin is manufactured in your body is in the pineal gland, which is deep inside the brain.[35] In other places such as the bone marrow and GI tract, melatonin is made in smaller amounts.[35] Melatonin may stop the spread of cancer, including breast, ovarian, colorectal, gastrointestinal, prostate and oral cancers.[36] Melatonin can act as an antioxidant, repairing damaged DNA in cells and has anti-inflammatory effect.[35] It suppresses cancer cell division and induces cancer cell death through a number of different pathways.[35] Melatonin also helps to interrupt cancer cells' ability to suppress anti-cell growth and cell death pathways; limits the ability of cancer cells to continue to divide indefinitely; interrupts cancer cell metabolism; and inhibits the growth of a blood supply to cancer tumors.[35] Melatonin also limits the ability of cancer cells to become invasive and helps to upregulate the immune system.[35] Melatonin can help improve cancer cells' receptivity of chemo while reducing its toxicity, even in cancers previously resistant to chemo medications, and can increase receptivity of both radiation and targeted therapies.[37,38] Because of these effects, melatonin has been proposed as a good supplementary treatment to amplify the effects of chemotherapy, radiation and targeted therapies.[36,38] Additionally, as melatonin is released in greater amounts in the evening to promote sleep, taking melatonin supplements can help reduce cancer-related sleep difficulties.[36]

Various mushrooms have anti-cancer properties that may prevent cancer as well as work to enhance traditional cancer treatments. Turkey Tail, Reishi, Shitake, and Maitake mushrooms activate the immune system, directly target tumor cells, and may reduce side effects from chemotherapy and radiation.[39,40] These mushrooms are safe to take in conjunction with traditional cancer treatments.[40] These mushrooms can be eaten or taken as supplements that contain the active compounds in the mushrooms. While my mom tried to take both Turkey Tail mushroom and AHCC (shitake mushroom) supplements, she was unable to tolerate them due to a food sensitivity to mushrooms.

Various teas have been reported as having anti-cancer properties and may be a useful addition to traditional cancer treatments. Essiac Tea has been used in Canada and the United States as an adjuvant cancer treatment. The recipe for Essiac tea, which contains the herbs Arctium lappa, Rumex acetosella, Ulmus rubra and Rheum officinale, has its origins in the Ojibwa tribe and was put into use by a nurse Rene Caisse in the 1920s in Canada.[41,42] Flor-essence contains watercress, blessed thistle, red clover and kelp in addition to the herbs in the original Essiac tea.[43] The herbs contained in Essiac tea have anti-oxidant and DNA-protective properties[41] and are proposed to activate the immune system and suppress tumor growth.[44] There is anecdotal evidence and one published case report[45] supporting the use of Essiac to improve quality of life and reduce mortality, but no large-scale clinical trials have been performed.[42] Essiac and Flor-essence are typically ingested 1-3 times a day on an empty stomach to minimize the likelihood of nausea, vomiting and diarrhea.[43]

Green tea (EGCG) consumption is associated with lower cancer risk and may help to improve survival time.[39] The EGCG compound in green tea has both antioxidant and thus anti-inflammatory effects and pro-oxidant effects, with the pro-oxidant effects playing an important role in cancer cell death and the cessation of cancer cell division.[46,47] Green tea reduces cancer cell growth and spread, reduces the formation of a tumor's blood supply, and induces cell death.[46]

Acupuncture

Acupuncture can be a safe and effective addition to cancer care.[c,48] Your hospital may even have an acupuncture center. Acupuncture stimulates regions on the body known as acupuncture points with thin needles that are inserted into these points. Acupuncture involves the placement of special needles into certain body points known as acupuncture points a few millimeters to a few centimeters into the skin; acupuncture can also involve manual manipulation of the needles, or application of heat or electric pulses.[26] Research suggests that acupuncture helps to balance nervous system activity, which may be how it is of benefit to overall well-being.[26] Some acupuncturists may also have additional training in Traditional Chinese Medicine, which works to restore balance in areas such as the environment, emotions, and diet through partial and systemic therapy, strengthening the body's ability to resist disease, eliminating pathogens and regulating emotions.[3] Traditional Chinese medicine can help to reduce the side effects of chemo and radiation and may help to limit tumor growth and thus increase survival.[3]

The benefits of acupuncture include reducing adverse effects of treatments such as nausea and vomiting, chemotherapy and radiation-related dry mouth, post-operative pain, cancer-related pain, insomnia, anxiety, and improving quality of life.[26,48] Acupuncture can help to reduce hot flashes that many women experience as a result of chemo. It can help to improve white blood cell count. It can help to reduce fatigue and the tingling and numbness in the hands and feet that some people experience post chemo. Acupuncture can improve the dry mouth that occurs with radiation treatment. Patients receiving palliative care may see all of the benefits noted above along with decreased physical and psychological distress and improved life satisfaction and mood.[48] You can use the National Certification Commission for Acupuncture and Oriental Medicine find-a-practitioner website to locate an acupuncturist near you (https://directory.nccaom.org/).[49]

Massage Therapy

Massage can help alleviate cancer symptoms and improve wellbeing.[50] People with cancer often experience pain and this pain can interfere with their physical health and emotional well-being.[51] It is estimated that about half of patients with cancer experience pain that ranges from mild to severe. Pain might be short-term due to treatment or surgery or can become chronic. While there are medications that can treat pain related to cancer, massage therapy may also be a useful treatment, without the side effects that come from medication. One study that combined the results of multiple studies found that massage therapy is effective in reducing pain intensity, severity, fatigue and anxiety.[50, 51] Massage is useful to decrease anxiety, depression, and pain in the short term.[26,50]

There are many different types of massage therapy techniques. Swedish massage is the most commonly practiced massage therapy in Europe and North America, which uses five different types of long, flowing strokes to decrease muscle tightness and stress.[26,50] Swedish massage is the most frequently studied type of massage with respect to cancer care.[26] Soft tissue release uses compression in a precise manner to decrease muscle spasm and scar tissue.[50] Foot reflexology is a specific type of massage to stimulate certain parts of the sole of the foot that are thought to relate to various organs or regions in the body.[26] Foot reflexology can induce reductions in chemotherapy-related peripheral neuropathy, and anxiety, depression, pain, and sleep quality.[52,53]

Patients who have cancer with lymph node involvement may find that lymphatic drainage and massage by a certified lymphaedema therapist helps to move lymph throughout the body and reduce the presence of lymphaedema. You can use the find a LANA-certified therapist feature on the Lymphology Association of North America's website https://www.clt-lana.org/search/therapists/.[54] These therapists are a range of health professionals from physical and occupational therapists to chiropractors, and licensed massage therapists. Because lymphatic drainage helps to remove toxins and boost immunity. this type of massage can be beneficial to anyone with cancer.[50]

Mind-Body Treatments

Mind-body techniques can be used to reduce anxiety and stress, and improve sleep quality and

> Mind-body techniques can reduce anxiety and stress, improve sleep and quality of life.

108

overall quality of life, particularly when paired with medication.[26] Mind-body modalities use the interaction between the mind and behavior in order to improve health and quality of life.[26] Mind-body techniques have the benefit of interrupting the cycle of cancer symptoms that can lead to emotional distress which leads to further cancer symptoms.[55] Reductions in overall stress can improve immune system functioning.[55] Examples of mind-body techniques are meditation, relaxation techniques, hypnotherapy, yoga, T'ai Chi, music therapy and Qi Gong.

Forest bathing is the act of spending time in nature, particularly forest environments. The act of forest bathing may can reduce production of the stress hormone cortisol, lower blood pressure and heart rate, and reduce the fight or flight response.[3] Forest bathing can promote the production of natural killer cells, promoting better immune system functioning.[3]

Mindfulness-based meditation is used to help a patient become an objective observer of their emotions, feelings and perceptions.[26] Mindfulness-based meditation helps to create a non-judgmental mindful state of conscious awareness.[26] This awareness without judgement can reduce the stress associated with symptoms related to cancer and cancer treatment, and improve sleep and health related quality of life. Regular practice of mindfulness meditation reduces cortisol secretion, decreases proinflammatory cytokines, and regulates the endocrine system.[3]

The mind-body techniques of sitting meditation and mindful movement are taught over a period of weeks. Yoga, T'ai chi and Qi Gong combine physical movement, postures, and breath control with meditation.[3] Some small trials have shown reduction of anxiety, depression, distress, and improved emotional well-being in patients with cancer who practice these techniques.[26] One recent meta-analysis that combined the effects of multiple studies examining T'ai Chi or Qi Gong on cancer symptoms found improvements in fatigue, sleep, depression, and quality of life and a potential to reduce pain.[56] Yoga interventions demonstrate sustained reductions in depression, anxiety, cancer-related fatigue, and sleep quality[57-59] and may help improve appetite and reduce chemo-related nausea and vomiting.[55] One organization, yoga4cancer (https://y4c.com/), can help you find a teacher trained in yoga practice for people living with cancer and has free online classes available as well.[60]

Hypnotherapy

Hypnosis has been used for pain management, insomnia, nausea and vomiting, boosting the immune system and general quality of life.[48] The guided imagery in hypnosis can alleviate chemo-related nausea and vomiting.

Relaxation training in hypnotherapy can reduce anxiety and nausea during chemo treatment and reduce the fight or flight response in the body, the level and frequency of anxiety, depression, chemo-induced hot flashes and prolonged nausea after chemo. They had less severe and less prolonged nausea at home. Hypnosis can improve quality of life. Patients who use hypnotherapy increase their immune system function with increases in percentage and activity of natural killer and T-cells responsible for a positive immune response, and decreased circulating levels of tumor necrosis factor, which is an inflammatory marker that is implicated in cancer. These chances can be seen even in patients receiving immunosuppressant treatments. Hypnosis can help children undergoing chemotherapy to control nausea and vomiting and reduce the amount of pain experienced.[48]

Aromatherapy

Aroma therapy uses essential oils to help manage the side effects of cancer and cancer treatment such as insomnia and nausea.[61] Essential oils can be inhaled by putting a drop or two on a tissue and breathing it, putting some drops into a diffuser that disperses the oil in the air, or via atomizing. Essential oils can be paired with a carrier oil and placed directly on the skin; however, cancer treatment may increase the skin's sensitivity and thus increase the likelihood of a skin reaction. When selecting an essential oil, look for one that is certified organic.[61] You should be mindful that some essential oils can reduce or enhance the effectiveness of certain medications; in particular, people with estrogen-dependent cancers should be mindful of this. Lavender, peppermint, and orange are common essential oils that can help support patients with cancer. Lavender creates a calming sensation to promote sleep. Peppermint can decrease nausea and vomiting. Peppermint oil can irritate the skin and may be better used in a diffuser; however, peppermint oil can be toxic to pets, so you may wish to skip this one if you have household pets. Orange oil can decrease anxiety and improve mood; however, if you are taking medication for anxiety or depression, this may increase the effects of this medication.[61] Working with an integrative physician or ND who is familiar with both your medications and the impact of essential oils will help you avoid any potential interactions.

If you decide you wish to pursue CAM, you may wish to consider what your goals are in order to best select which treatments are best. If you wish to pursue this as an adjuvant treatment for your cancer, it would be best to start with an integrative physician or ND who specializes in cancer care. Your health insurance may even cover this. From there, have a realistic conversation about your financial situation and what you can afford. The ND or integrative physician could work with you to help prioritize which treatments would be the best for you to pursue. If your goal is to reduce side effects, then perhaps a single modality such as acupuncture or mindfulness techniques would be a good choice. There are many free resources in the area of mindfulness on the internet, that would promote wellbeing.

❖❖❖❖❖❖❖❖❖❖❖❖❖❖❖❖❖❖❖

Notes and Questions

❖❖❖❖❖❖❖❖❖❖❖❖❖❖❖❖❖❖❖

Chapter 7 Exercise

The association of lower rates of cancer with higher rates of exercise has been known since the 1940s.[1] Exercise is also an important component in cancer treatment. Exercise is any type of planned, structured repetitive movement.[2] According to the American Heart Association physical inactivity is one of the biggest health risk factors with only approximately 25% of men, and approximately 20% of women and children meeting current exercise guidelines.[3,4] Better cardiorespiratory fitness is associated with decreased cancer diagnoses and mortality.[5] Physical activity has a role in the prevention and management of chronic diseases such as cancer.[6] Together, physical activity, weight loss and healthy diet can help to improve physical functioning and reduce mobility disability.

My mom was very active in middle age and through older adulthood. She took up running in her 50s and learned to ski in her 60s. Having played tennis on her high school team, she loved racket sports and started to play pickleball in her 70s. Mom ran several times a week-she even ran the Purple Strides 5K that raises money for pancreatic cancer in the middle of her chemo treatments, stopping to walk only once because her chemo made her sensitive to the cold and she needed to catch her breath. When the weather turned too cold in the winter months for her to tolerate outside exercise paired with chemo, I set up her bike on my indoor trainer and gave her an old laptop so she could watch movies while biking in her basement. She skied with a friend that she had met in her learn-to-ski class at least once a week and I would drive my daughters with their snowboards to meet them. They would happily ride the lifts together - I could hear their laughter while I sat by the firepit grading student papers and editing my own research manuscripts. My mom's pickleball group had an online meet up and mom would sign up for any slot she could. She would sit out a set if she was tired but loved just getting out there and playing. Not only was mom getting the benefits of exercise, but also the benefits of social connections.

Types of Exercise

The American College of Sports Medicine recommendations for cancer prevention are that all adults engage in 150-300 minutes a week of moderate or 75-150 minutes a week of vigorous aerobic exercise that is spread throughout the week. Additional recommendations include at least two days a week of strength training and daily flexibility exercises.[7] The American College of Sports Medicine states that exercise is safe for patients with cancer and cancer survivors and that the exercise guidelines for adults should be followed with the addition of balance exercises.[8]

They note that some specific precautions might need to be taken for those with lymphedema, peripheral neuropathies, breast reconstruction, and those with central lines or ostomies.[8] Exercise has

American College of Sports Medicine states: "exercise is safe for patients with cancer and cancer survivors"

not been found to cause or increase the progression of lymphaedema.[9] Exercise training can be broken up into smaller bouts of at least 10 minutes throughout the day. Individuals with chronic health conditions such as cancer or disabilities who are not able to meet these guidelines should engage in regular physical activity according to their abilities. In other words, some exercise is better than no exercise. If you are unable to meet these exercise guidelines, consulting a physical therapist can help you optimize your exercise time to get the maximum benefit.[7]

Aerobic exercise is exercise that primarily promotes cardiovascular endurance (your heart and lungs) by increasing your breathing and heart rate, typically through the continuous use of large muscle groups.[2,8] Common forms of aerobic exercise include walking, running, cycling, and swimming.

Resistance, or strength-training, primarily targets the musculoskeletal system (your muscles and bones). Resistance training moves the body against some form of external resistance such as body weight (as in the case of a pushup), resistance bands, or dumbbells.[2] Resistance training should work all major muscle groups of the body to increase the quality, size, and strength of a muscle as well as muscle power, which is the ability to generate force quickly. Muscle power is important for tasks such as walking up a flight of stairs, walking quickly, or preventing a loss of balance that could result in a fall. Flexibility training can maintain or increase the range of motion of all joints through activities such as stretching, yoga, or T'ai Chi.

Figure 7.1 Modified Borg Rating of Perceived Exertion[12]

0	Rest
1	Really Easy
2	Easy
3	Moderate
4	Sort of Hard
5	Hard
6	
7	Really Hard
8	
9	Extremely Hard
10	Exhausted

Moderate intensity exercise is defined as exercise that is "somewhat hard" to "hard." Vigorous intensity is defined as exercising at an intensity that is "hard" to "very hard." While physical therapists and other health care professionals typically use heart rate to help measure exercise intensity, this can be measured in more simple ways. One is through the use of the Talk Test. If you are able to comfortably talk but not sing while exercising, then you are working at moderate intensity.[10,11] If you can speak, but no more than a sentence, then you are exercising at vigorous intensity.[10] Another way is through using the modified Borg scale (Figure 7.1) in which rating your exercise as 5-6/10 is moderate and 7/10 is vigorous.[12,13]

Cancer Prevention

Exercise decreases the number of new cases of cancer each year.[14] An estimated 35% of 7 million cancer deaths each year are lifestyle related.[6,15] There is strong evidence in favor of exercise reducing the risk of

> The greater level of physical activity, the greater the decrease in risk from all cancer mortality.

bladder, breast, colon, endometrial, esophageal, adenocarcinoma, renal and gastric cancers, with reductions ranging from 10 to 20%.[6,16] Greater volumes of physical activity (frequency of activity multiplied by the length of time) reduce cancer risk.[6] Physical activity can be formal activity such as labor-intensive work activities or exercise or can be more informal such as the accumulation of activity through household chores or walking your dog(s). The reduction in body mass index, that may result from exercise, can lower the risk of cancer particularly with respect to breast, colon, pancreatic, prostate, endometrial, ovarian, and lung cancers.[15]

Physical activity improves immune system functioning through lowering inflammatory markers, insulin growth factor (IGF-1), leptin, and insulin. Insulin and IGF-1 play a role in cancer by promoting cell growth and inhibiting cell death.[8,15,17] Inflammation is linked to a variety of chronic diseases including cancer and is also linked to higher body mass index. Inflammation may inhibit healthy cell growth and promote the progression of damaged cell growth. Exercise helps to increase levels and activity of immune cells such as T cells, natural killer cells, and neutrophils. While these increases are short-lived, regular moderate-to-vigorous exercise may help to create a cumulative effect of these immune system increases.[15,18]

While emphasis is on moderate- to vigorous-intensity exercise, any increase in physical activity will be of benefit. This is particularly true for older adults, who are at risk greater risk for cancer and who may be cancer survivors.[1] The research is clear that the greater level of physical activity, the greater the decrease in risk from all cancer mortality.

Prehabilitation

Prehabilitation, or physical rehabilitation prior to cancer surgery or treatment, can improve overall outcomes such as reduced cancer symptom burden and improved survival.[19] Prehabilitation may help to improve aerobic capacity so that exercise can continue during and after treatment and should be started as soon as possible.[8] If you are new to exercise, a program of lower intensity can increase the likelihood that you will stick with the exercises.[20] Continuation of exercise will promote your functional capacity and can boost your immune system functioning.[20] Prehabilitation increases the chances that you will stay with your exercise program and improves tolerance for cancer treatments.[9] Prehabilitation may improve treatment outcomes by improving lung function, reducing post-operative complications, reducing hospital length of stay and potentially changing the biology of your tumor or increasing its likelihood to respond to treatment.[21,22] A high-intensity prehabilitation program is demonstrated to be safe and improves function after surgery and during and after other cancer treatments.[23] A recommended six to eight weeks of prehabilitation represents a length of time to ensure efficacy of exercise interventions while not delaying cancer treatment for an unacceptable length of time. However, some prehabilitation is better than none; try to get some physical therapy prior to starting treatment.[22] A high-intensity interval training program - periods of intense exercise interspersed with rest periods - is particularly useful in situations where there is a short window of time between diagnosis and surgery or treatment.[19]

Exercise during Cancer Treatment

Exercise is safe, beneficial, and feasible for adults and also children with cancer.[9,24] Research shows that those who do not exercise while undergoing cancer treatment have poorer physical functioning and quality of life and greater psychological distress.[2] Exercise impacts the bodies and minds of children by reducing body mass and fat, fatigue and depression, and improving physical fitness.[8,24] While declines in physical fitness and function during chemotherapy treatment is documented, this can be minimized with a progressive program of exercise. Exercise type can range from aerobic exercise, aerobic paired with progressive resistance (strength) training, yoga, dance, and progressive resistive exercise.[9] Even walking three to four days a week at a slower speed can prevent some typical decline and promote function.[8] Choose the exercise that you are most likely to do!

Exercise improves mental health, including anxiety, quality of life, and mood.[8,18,25-27] Both resistance and aerobic training can reduce the emotional symptom

> **Exercise improves mental health and should be considered a first-line choice of treatment when undergoing cancer therapies.**

burden of cancer such as feeling sad or irritable.[28] As a result, we should consider exercise to be a first-line choice of treatment for patients undergoing cancer therapies. Even for patients with metastatic lung cancer with reduced aerobic capacity, modifying exercise frequency and length helped to maximize physical function.[29] It might be hard to modify activities you were once able to do with ease, but it is important to keep moving. Walking can be a convenient form of exercise as it is easy to increase or decrease the length of time and your walking speed according to how you are feeling. You could even break your walking into smaller, more frequent bouts to help you maintain your functional level.[29]

The reduction of systemic inflammation, improved metabolism, and reduced fat tissue seen with exercise has many positive impacts. These include DNA repair within cells; decreased systemic stress; reduced cancer cell division and increase cancer cell death; reduced blood supply to the tumors; and enhanced immune system functioning.[30] Exercise can help level out sex hormones, which are implicated in some cancers.[14,18] Exercise positively impacts blood cell numbers, particularly immune cells.[8,24] Exercise may increase the effectiveness of anti-cancer treatments, particularly immunotherapy, by allowing the tumor to be more receptive to treatment.[2,14,18] Exercise can also promote the invasion of immune cells into the cancer tumor.[14] Exercise, particularly interval training, can boost the number and function of a type of white blood cell called neutrophils, which can lower your risk of infection during cancer treatment.[18] It is also associated with a slowing of tumor growth that is associated with improved immune system functioning.[14]

Regular exercise can help you to counteract both the impact of and the treatment for your cancer.[23] Exercise can help to reduce cancer-related pain[26] and treatment side effects such as decreased bone density, neuropathy, heart disease, and cancer-related fatigue.[2,8,18] Deconditioning can occur during cancer treatment.[15] Because aerobic exercise and strength training improve cardiovascular endurance and muscle strength, fatigue and weakness related to cancer treatment will be improved by these forms of exercise. Aerobic exercise and strength training will also improve muscle mass (also known as lean or fat free mass) and bone mass while decreasing fat mass, BMI and waist circumference.[15]

Chemotherapy-related toxicity and brain fog are also reduced through exercise.[18] Exercise helps to reduce treatment side effects such as swelling, pain, and heart and lung issues.[2,23,25] Because survivors might experience persistent side effects from either the cancer or the treatment, exercise might be helpful to treat this.[2] Exercise improves the flow of lymphatic fluid which improves your immune system functioning.[2]

Cachexia is a continuous depletion of skeletal muscle mass sometimes accompanied by a reduction of fat mass which can lead to progressive decline in physical functioning.[31] If you lose muscle mass, you lose strength, and reduce your functional abilities. Cancer-related cachexia cannot be reversed with nutritional support. Your total daily energy expenditure is comprised of your resting expenditure, your expenditure during physical activity, and the thermogenic effect of the food you consumed. Cachexia is the result of one, or a combination of, not eating or exercising enough, inflammation, and the energy needs of your tumor.[31] Because exercise can help increase anti-inflammatory markers in your blood stream, it can help to decrease the muscle wasting seen with cachexia.[31]

The loss of muscle mass seen with cancer treatment, a sedentary lifestyle, and malnutrition due to cancer and cancer treatment can impact your body's ability to process chemo.[32] Regular exercise can decrease the risk of experiencing toxic effects of chemo or immunotherapy.[32] Exercise may help you remain on your current chemo regimen or stay in a clinical trial.

When Cancer Treatment Ends

People who exercise regularly have a lower risk of cancer recurrence, which may be due to the reduction of inflammatory markers.[2,26] Despite this, research shows that people undergoing cancer as well as those who are cancer survivors, have lower levels of physical activity than those who have never had cancer.[33] Because exercise helps to improve cardiovascular health and muscle mass, it decreases your likelihood of experiencing additional health issues

> Exercise will improve your overall health and well-being so that you can live your life

when treatment ends.[21] Exercise will improve your overall health and well-being so that you can live your life.[21]

If you are receiving hospice services, exercise is still appropriate for you. Exercise can help you maintain your independence and mobility and help boost your mood.[23] If you have not had a physical therapist referred as part of your hospice team, ask the hospice nurse assigned to your case.

Mortality

Physical activity is important in prevention of cancer, but it can also provide health benefits after cancer diagnosis. People who exercise regularly have a lower risk of cancer-specific mortality and a decreased risk of dying from any cause.[2,16,18,34] Higher pre-diagnosis and post-diagnosis exercise levels collectively improve survival outcomes for at least 11 different cancers.[34] Even if you weren't very active before your cancer diagnosis, increasing your activity levels to the suggested 150 minutes of moderate activity a week will provide you the benefits of increased survival.[35] This provides strong evidence that exercise should be included in any cancer rehabilitation program. Death from cardiovascular disease among cancer survivors is also reduced with greater levels of exercise; maintaining or increasing exercise levels should be promoted after cancer treatment ends.[34]

Physical activity can help improve muscle strength, aerobic capacity and quality of life and is implicated in the survival of breast, colon, and prostate cancers.[2,18,36] One study found that older adults meeting the recommendations of at least two days a week of strength training had 46% lower odds of all-cause mortality.[37]

Physical functioning can be maintained with exercise, which is particularly important for patients with cancer. In one study, overall physical functioning was associated with lower all-cause mortality and a 50% reduction in the risk of premature death.[15] Faster walking speed is also associated with better median survival rates and decreased premature death.[15]

Getting Started with Exercise

So now that you can appreciate the value of physical activity, let's look at how you get started. Models of care have been developed to provide access to physical therapists, but these are unfortunately not used widely. This demonstrates a need for more precise guidelines for referral to physical therapy.[38,39] Poor care coordination is another barrier to providing physical activity counseling.[4] For example, one survey of patients with multiple myeloma found that less than half received recommendations about exercise from a health care professional, less than 15% were referred to physical therapy by their oncologist, with another 5% referred to physical therapy if they asked their oncologist.[40] If every health discipline expects another discipline to discuss physical activity with you, the likelihood of you receiving exercise information is low. The oncologist's office is typically the central coordinator of cancer care, but if the oncologist does not ask about your physical activity level, then a referral to a physical therapist is unlikely.[4] The oncology team may not have an understanding of the role of exercise in cancer care; research indicates that healthcare providers worry about increasing psychological stress or causing patients to overexert themselves.[41] However, proper exercise counseling results in lower symptom burden and improvements in overall health.[42] A physical therapist-led exercise assessment and counseling significantly improves fatigue, psychological distress, mental health, overall health ratings, physical health, and appetite.

Because physical therapists are trained to conduct exercise testing; provide physical activity counseling; and prescribe exercise to their patients, you should have a referral to a physical therapist either for prehabilitation prior to surgery and/or the start of your other cancer treatments, or for exercise to cope during and after treatment.[4] Additionally, health outcomes are enhanced with supervised exercise sessions and increase the likelihood that you will regularly perform exercise.[9] If you are not offered physical therapy, you should ask your oncologist. You can also use the American Physical Therapy Association's "Find-a-PT" function https://www.choosept.com/resources/choose.aspx to locate one yourself.

People with cancer are more likely to exercise if they expect improvements in physical and mental health and symptoms; if they are independent; and if they have social support.[23] People with cancer are less likely to exercise if they are fearful of exercise, if they have challenges adapting to diagnosis, poor prognosis, multiple other health issues, a current sedentary lifestyle, or poor access to exercise programs.[23] Your oncologist should ask you about your current physical activity level and the types of exercise you like to do. You can also refer yourself to outpatient physical therapy without a doctor's prescription, although your insurance may require a referral.

While vigorous exercise is touted as the best way to improve longevity,[43] you should feel confident that some physical activity is better than no physical activity. If you're unable to participate in vigorous physical activity, participate in moderate physical activity and take breaks when needed. This will still promote your overall health and longevity.

Regardless of where you are on your journey, you should consider consulting with a physical therapist, who can work with you to find the right combination of strength and aerobic training at the right dosage and intensity so that you can maintain or improve your function. Because physical therapists are exercise and movement specialists, you can be confident that the information you receive is accurate. At one point during my mom's treatment, a nurse scolded her for exercising and told her that she needed to rest to make her heart stronger. As a physical therapist, I can assure you that since your heart is a muscle, you need exercise to make it stronger.

A physical therapist can make sure to prescribe you exercises that are safe for you given your cancer and any other health issues you might have whether they are from cancer like bone metastases or things like high blood pressure. Your physical therapist can monitor your blood pressure, heart rate, and oxygen saturation during your physical therapy sessions to make sure they prescribe a program tailored to you. Bodies were meant to move, yours included. There is no better time than right now to get started on an exercise program.

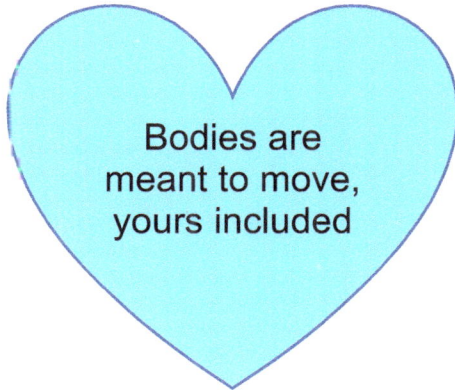

Bodies are meant to move, yours included

❖ ❖ ❖ ❖ ❖ ❖ ❖ ❖ ❖ ❖ ❖ ❖ ❖ ❖ ❖ ❖ ❖ ❖
Notes and Questions
❖ ❖ ❖ ❖ ❖ ❖ ❖ ❖ ❖ ❖ ❖ ❖ ❖ ❖ ❖ ❖ ❖ ❖

Chapter 8 Nutrition

One of the most challenging areas to navigate after a cancer diagnosis is in the area of nutrition. There are so many different dietary approaches for patients with cancer that it can seem overwhelming to select an appropriate one. After my mom was diagnosed, we read books that advocated juicing, some that advocated smoothies, others that talked about a whole-food, plant-based diet. While I read about these different approaches, my mom received advice from her oncology team to eat anything she wanted to keep weight on - after all, she had a GI cancer and was undergoing chemotherapy. The team's feeling was that it didn't matter what she ate as long as she was eating. Given that there is a Food as Medicine movement with hospitals such as Loma Linda University offering residents specialty training in this area, I knew that there were other health professionals who disagreed with this approach.[1] Both of us were determined to make dietary adjustments after reading the research on the association between diet and cancer. But which dietary approach should you choose?

In this chapter, I will review a few dietary practices so that you can gain a basic understanding of what each approach entails. This will provide you with some information to choose a dietary approach to further investigate or will give you an idea of different approaches to discuss with your registered dietician, integrative physician, or physical therapist. It is my belief that the best dietary practice to select is the one that will be the easiest to follow. Shifts in dietary practices should feel supportive of your overall health instead of causing you stress. If you select one way to eat and it does not seem to be working for you, then

> **The best dietary practice to select is the one that will be the easiest to follow.**

change it. The most important thing is that you are eating whole, unprocessed foods that will support your quest to make your body as inhospitable to cancer as possible. This chapter will discuss a whole-foods, plant-based approach, the Mediterranean Diet, the Keto diet, and intermittent fasting.

Whole Foods, Plant-based Approach

Vegetarian and vegan diets are associated with decreased cancer incidence and[2] fruit and vegetable intake is associated with a decreased risk of cancer mortality.[3] Data from the China Study conducted in the 1970s notes a significantly decreased intake of fat and protein in people living in rural China as compared to Western diets, and an increased intake in fiber typical of a plant-based diet were associated with decreased cancer rates.[4] Plant-based foods are the only sources of dietary fiber and protein intake in rural Chinese, not animal sources.[4] Whole foods, plant-based (WFPB) diets can play an important role in cancer prevention and treatment. High-fiber, low-fat diets are associated with lower rates of colorectal cancers and reducing dietary fat can improve outcomes for patients with breast cancer.[5,6] A WFPB diet is associated with lower mortality rates in the general population.[7]

Intake of animal protein is associated with increased mortality from any cause, heart disease, and cancer.[8] Reducing protein intake has been proposed as a way to prevent and treat cancer.[9] Protein intake influences all stages of cancer development. Protein can initiate tumor development through DNA damage and transport of cancer-causing chemicals.[10] In the promotion stage, increased protein intake is associated with increased levels of growth hormone and IGF-1; increase division of mutated cancer cells; faster cell metabolism that fuels cancer cell division; and decreased immune system functioning, particularly through decreases in natural killer cells.[8,10,11] Low-protein diets, particularly diets initiated prior to older adulthood, decrease the risk of

> **Reducing protein intake has been proposed as a way to prevent and treat cancer.**

tumor development, even in liver tumors that are due to a viral cause.[12] Vegetarians and vegans, while replacing animal-based protein with plant-based proteins, tend to consume lower overall levels of protein.[13] Intake of plant-based protein is associated with lower mortality from any cause including cardiovascular disease.[8] Consuming plant-based protein reduces risk for many diseases, including cancer.[14] It makes sense to explore a WFPB diet for a potential dietary shift.

Advocates of the WFPB approach cite evidence that nutritional imbalances promote chronic diseases such as cancer and reversing these imbalances with a WFPB approach can halt and reverse disease.[10,15] It is possible to have the majority of your nutritional needs met through the WFPB diet. The one exception is vitamin B12, which is typically found in animal sources. B12 is readily available in supplement form. Adherence to lifestyle changes that included WFPB eating, exercise, stress reduction and social support were found to reduce prostate specific antigen levels, a marker for prostate cancer, and inhibit tumor growth in men with prostate cancer, with those who followed these changes more closely having improved scores.[16-18] Even more exciting was the influence at the level of over 500 genes; protective genes were switched on and cancer promoting genes were switched off after 3 months of these changes.[17] The lifestyle changes you have been reading about in this book make a difference even in a short period of time! In addition to decreased protein consumption, non-meat eaters also tend to consume less sugar, alcohol, and fried foods.[13] If you are not ready to go completely plant-based, replacing a portion of the protein from meat sources in your diet with WFPB meals and decreasing your intake of sugar, fried foods, and alcohol can still make an impact on your diet. A high-quality diet that emphasizes fruits, vegetables, whole grains and legumes can help improve your overall health.[19]

The Mediterranean Diet

The Mediterranean Diet (MedDiet) is one way of eating that may be a middle ground between going completely plant-based and staying with the standard American diet (SAD). The MedDiet emphasizes whole foods including whole grains, plant-based foods such as vegetables, fruits, nuts, seeds, and legumes, fish and poultry, extra virgin olive oil, and low- or non-fat dairy.[20] Another feature of the MedDIET is the reduction in or elimination of red meat, processed foods, and sugary foods and beverages.[20] This diet can be viewed as a lifestyle intervention because it also emphasizes social meals and exercise, which are also important to people with cancer.[20,21]

Overall mortality and cancer mortality is reduced in those who adhere to the MedDiet.[22,23] Because this diet is high in plant protein and in lean proteins such as fish, it may be useful to both decrease cancer risk and can be an important intervention once diagnosed

> **The Mediterranean diet is high in plant proteins and lean proteins, such as fish.**

with cancer.[24,25] The MedDiet has many health benefits for people diagnosed with cancer.[19,26] This diet can decrease oxidative stress which is associated with both cancer initiation and progression. Blood clot risk is decreased; people with cancer are at increased risk for clots.[24] The MedDiet has a high fiber content, which helps to reduce the absorption of cancer-causing chemicals in the small intestine and promotes the excretion of excess estrogen in the stool.[24] The hormones IGF-1, estrogen and testosterone are reduced in people adhering to this diet, reducing the risk of tumor growth.[24] Foods in the MedDiet such as tomatoes, onions, garlic, pumpkin, and carrots reduce risk for cancer and reduce inflammation that can promote cancer growth.[27] Chronic pain can be a feature of cancer and cancer treatment. Chemical compounds found in nuts, salmon, extra virgin olive oil, rosemary, sage, olives, red wine all help to reduce chronic pain.[28,29] Additionally, muscle mass and bone density are preserved with the MedDiet; both muscle mass and bone density are often reduced from cancer and cancer treatment.[30-32] Cancer-related fatigue is reduced and quality of life is increased in those who adhere to the MedDiet.[33]

Because this diet is non-restrictive and does not require special food, it may be easier to follow for someone undergoing cancer treatment. This diet may be easier to integrate into regular meal planning for families. MedDiet recipes are readily available online.

The Ketogenic Diet

The ketogenic (keto) diet refers to eating a high-fat, low carbohydrate diet. The premise for the usefulness of this diet for people living with cancer is that cancer relies on the sugar from the breakdown of carbohydrates to survive and divide. In the absence of carbohydrates, the liver breaks down fatty acids for energy. The resultant ketone bodies are unable to be used by the cancer cells

> The ketogenic diet is a high-fat, low carbohydrate diet. Removing carbohydrates limits sugar that cancer cells use as fuel to survive and divide.

for fuel. Some patients may have concerns about this diet, because of the protein that is consumed, due to the association of protein with risk of cancer and mortality.[14] A typical ratio for this diet is three to four fats for every one carbohydrate/protein, so that the diet is 90% fat, 8% protein, and 2% carbohydrate.[34,35] This amount of protein is not particularly high; the MedDiet typically have between 5-25% of the diet coming from protein.[36] Because of the limited protein intake, some people have long-term difficulties in following this dietary plan. Suggestions in the literature look to a 2:1 fat to carbohydrate/protein ratio as still being anticancer, but easier to follow.[35] Cookbooks and internet sources of recipes can also help to support patients who wish to implement this diet.[35]

The thought behind the usefulness of this diet as an anti-cancer modality is that by depriving the cancer cells of the sugar they need for energy, the cancer cells are stressed and become more receptive to chemotherapy and radiation.[34,37] While clinical trials indicate that some cancers such as gliomas cannot use ketone bodies (the byproducts of protein) for energy, other trials such as breast cancer indicate that some cancer cells can use ketone bodies.[35] So while the keto diet does have anti-cancer properties, it may not solely be from depriving cancer cells of a needed energy source.

Some case studies and clinical trials have reported reduced tumor progression in patients following the keto diet.[35] This may be due to boosting the immune system;[38] the documented interruption of the formation of a blood supply to tumors in mouse models;[39] or alterations in gene expression in response to this diet.[40] Additionally, improvements in blood glucose and cholesterol levels and energy in patients with cancer have been reported after following this diet.[35] The reduction in blood sugar is accompanied by a reduction in IGF-1, which reduces the growth of cancer cells.[35] The lower protein levels of the keto diet downregulate essential amino acids, which may also contribute to the anti-cancer properties of this diet.[35] Because of the composition of this diet, consulting with your healthcare team is important to ensure you are getting all of the vitamins and minerals you need.[35] Despite the difficulties that some people may experience adhering to the keto diet, it does hold promise for use with cancer therapy to increase the cancer's response to this therapy.[41]

Intermittent Fasting

Intermittent fasting (IF) is a nutritional approach that could be used in conjunction with any of the methods of eating above or on its own without any other dietary changes. IF is a style of eating in which food is not consumed for an extended period of time. This fasting might occur during each day where fasting might occur for periods of 10-16 consecutive hours, with food consumed during the non-fasting window.[42] The advantage of this type of fasting is that for a sizeable portion of the fast, the individual is sleeping. Other

> **Intermittent fasting is a style of eating in which food is not consumed for an extended period of time.**

fasts might occur for one or two days a week, where an individual consumes food normally on non-fasting days and has one or two 24-hour cycles in which no food is consumed.[42] IF diets have reduced tumor occurrence, tumor progression, mortality, and chemotherapy toxicity in laboratory animals.[42] It is thought that the reduction in body weight associated with IF may decrease the risk of the cancers associated with overweight and obesity.[42] In addition to reducing body mass, IF reduces markers such as fasting glucose and IGF-1, both of which are associated with cancer as well as C-reactive protein, an inflammatory marker.[42,43] This dietary practice promotes the clearing out of damaged cells, suppresses cancer cell spread, and promotes preferential response of cancer cells to chemotherapy and radiation.[44,45] IF also reduces chemotherapy side effects such as gastrointestinal upset, exhaustion, and weakness and can prevent low red blood cell and platelet counts.[45]. Additionally, the caloric restriction paired with decreased protein intake reduces growth hormone and IGF-1 levels; these reductions are associated with decreased cancer incidence.[14]

Taking Stock of Your Diet

So how to choose what path to take with your nutrition? The first thing you might consider is tracking what foods you eat across a week. How many servings of fruits and vegetables do you eat each week? The recommendations are to consume 5-7 servings per day, but most Americans only consume 1-2 servings each day.[46] The greater the number of fruits and vegetables you are eating, the greater the reduction of inflammation in your body.[47] If you aren't hitting at least 5 servings, this might be a good place to start. Try to increase your intake by gradually increasing your servings. Maybe try making a smoothie for breakfast-spinach and kale blend easily into fruits smoothies without changing its taste.

How much added sugar is in your diet? The average American consumes 22 teaspoons of sugar every day.[48] Candy, soft drinks, and processed foods can be sources of sugar that are easily eliminated. Are you snacking on foods like chips that are ultra-processed and have high trans fats? Trans fats are associated with increased inflammation. Are you eating fast food or frozen prepared dinners regularly?

These can be sources of trans fats and sodium that will not promote overall wellness.

You might find that your diet is lacking in fruits and vegetables and is laden with added sugar, trans fats, and sodium. Starting by addressing these areas is a solid first step promoting overall wellness so that you can focus on having a high quality of life while you treat your cancer. It may be easier to make smaller changes by reducing fast food and soft drinks and increasing the number of plant-based foods you eat versus jumping into IF or the MEDdiet. If you want to do a complete overhaul of your diet all at once, this is great. Just remember that the best changes are the ones you can maintain. If you are just starting, making one small change and adding additional changes as you go can help you create long-term healthy habits.

❖❖❖❖❖❖❖❖❖❖❖❖❖❖❖❖❖❖
Notes and Questions
❖❖❖❖❖❖❖❖❖❖❖❖❖❖❖❖❖❖

Chapter 9 Getting Doctors to See the Whole You

It is my hope that this book provides you with foundational information so that you can hit the ground running in getting the best treatment for your cancer. This book is not an exhaustive review of all of the published literature that is out there, but you can use the basic information to do additional research for a deeper dive into what might be best for you given your type of cancer, your stage of cancer, your personal genetics and the genetics of your tumor.

Once you have this information and you have selected your medical team, you will want them to see you as a person who happens to have cancer. You are not your cancer. When my mom was diagnosed and in subsequent appointments

> You are not your cancer

with her oncologist and the medical opinions she had afterwards, she always made sure to tell them about herself. She told them that she was a retired teacher who had taught every grade from preschool through high school. She let them know how important it was that she help homeschool my children until they were at least finished 8th grade. She told them that she skied twice a week in the winter and played in a pickleball league year-round and that she was disappointed that the 5-FU pump kept her from running in the Hot Chocolate 5K. She wanted them to know she had friends from every part of her life with whom she wanted to spend meaningful time. Her healthcare team had a clear picture of who she was - an active, loved human being who was dealt a bad hand of cancer and who was not going to let cancer get in the way of her living her best life. My mom had a motto, "I am not dying today," and each day she proved that to be true.

One friend upon diagnosis brought a picture of her young daughter in with her to her first appointment and said that this is what she wanted to live for - the message being the oncologist needed to get on board with that. Another friend impressed upon the oncologist that travel was of the utmost importance and she would be working her treatments around her travel schedule. Box 9.1 provides examples of information you might want to provide your oncologist.

When entering into a patient-doctor relationship with your doctor, there may be other people who see the whole you who you would like to weigh in on decision making. You may want a shared decision-making relationship with your physician, but you might also want your family, friends, or spiritual/religious advisors to provide an opinion as well.[1] These opinions might not be medically informed but may help give you reassurance since you are ultimately known better by your social support network than your oncologist. My mom, brother, and I always discussed treatment options together. I always acknowledged that I had a hard time not just taking charge with my own healthcare background, but that ultimately, any decision was my mom's to make as she knew her body best. If she had told me in November 2017 that she did not want to even try chemotherapy, I would have accepted that no matter how hard it was.

This brings us to an issue in being seen for the whole you, which is the issue of patient preference. There may be varying opinions between oncologists as to whether oncologist expertise or patient preference should be the main factor in making cancer decisions. Decisions impact all areas of your life-finances, side effects, transportation, and logistics of treatment. Oncologists may assume they understand your preferences but may also not ask about them.[1] You want an oncologist who will engage with you at the level of your preferences and who is willing to honor those preferences. If you feel your oncologist does not understand your preferences, then tell them what your preferences are.

Your oncologist, when seeing you for the person that you are will help present treatment decisions that pair evidence-based cancer treatment with what you are identifying as your goals and will balance this against the value of cancer treatments. However, oncologists have differing views on the meaning of the word value[2]. The majority of oncologists will look at patients' and care givers' quality of life.[2] Will the treatment be a burden? Does the literature say there is statistically significant survival, but that survival time is one month, and that month will be fraught with side effects? An oncologist looking at quality of life will discuss these questions with you. Quality of life also includes pain control and mental health.[2] Oncologists might discuss the amount of time spent in medical care versus patients being able to live their lives as an element of value.[2] My mom's oncologist was very good at focusing on skipping treatments so that she felt well enough for her 50th college reunion and when our family visited from Germany. He said to her if it shortened her life by a few days, he felt they could agree that it was worth it-and they did agree on that point. Oncologists may also prioritize a patient-centric view of value and may discuss with you how the time and financial costs and health benefits could affect a patient directly. They may discuss how two drugs have similar efficacy, but that one is substantially less expensive or requires less frequent infusions.[2] When my mom and I were exploring the Care Oncology Clinic protocol mentioned in chapter 6, the oncologist talked about the cost of consulting with them as it wasn't covered by insurance and was worried about the financial implications. He also tried to get her into the hospital health system for her vitamin C infusions so they would be covered by insurance-although the consult fee to get into that program paired with the waiting list made continuing with our out-of-pocket payment the better plan in the end. While we knew that we could afford to pursue these options, I very much appreciated that he was aware of insurance constraints.

Box 9.1 Important Information to Consider and Tell Your Oncologist

Do you have a strong social support network? Who can you count on for things like transportation to treatments?

Do you live alone or with someone?

Are you a parent? How old are your children?

Do you hope to become a parent?

Are you a caregiver for a family member?

Are you employed? How demanding is your job physically or mentally? How many hours do you work a week? Is your job flexible?

What are your hobbies?

What is your physical activity level like? What kinds of exercise do you typically do?

Do you volunteer for any organizations? What kind of service do you perform?

How do you like to spend your free time?

Your oncologist might define value in terms of a more holistic approach to patient care where a patient entering a health system for cancer already has access to physical therapists and registered dieticians while engaging in their standard cancer care.[2] This was one area where I wished our hospital system was better. Our third opinion hospital seemed to have a much more integrated approach in terms of access to services, but the time it would have taken to go for cancer care would have been a burden. My mom was only offered access to a more holistic approach in the last few months of her life; it might have made a bigger impact if offered earlier.

Some oncologists feel that a discussion of cost may need to come first in the discussion of treatment and others feel that patients' preferences should be discussed prior to discussing treatment cost.[2] When it comes to finances of affording your cancer care, this may be left to the oncologist to discuss, or the oncologist may leave this to a social worker or financial advisor from the hospital would step in to help. Because of the wide range of opinions on what constitutes value, you should talk to your oncologist about what their own view is in terms of selecting chemotherapy regimens. Find out how aware are the oncologist is of the costs of each medication and how much insurance or other granting organizations will pay versus how much you will pay. If you need help affording a medication, ask to meet with a social worker. Also look at cancer-specific foundations for programs that may help with affordability. Finally there are granting organizations such as the PAN Foundation https://www.panfoundation.org/ that can help you afford your medications.[3] In our own experience, the cost of care was never discussed with my mom and I, despite the fact that patients with Medicare are responsible for 20% of cost of an infused medication, which is a significant amount.

If your oncologist can see you for the whole you, then they will provide you with patient-centered care, which is essential for your well-being. Patient-centered care means that your needs, preferences, values and autonomy and independence will be respected.[4] It means you will participate in a partnership with the oncologist to share decision making.[4] If your oncologist comes in with a paternalistic view that they know what is best for you and should make all of the decisions,[4] then refer back to chapter 5 and get that second opinion. Decide for yourself whether you want an informed decision-making relationship in which your oncologist gives you all the information to make a decision or a shared decision-making relationship in which you and your oncologist negotiate toward treatment decisions.[4] You want a relationship in which you are empowered to make decisions. The paternalistic view of our first oncologist consult is what drove us to the shared decision-making oncologist that treated my mom throughout her cancer.

The book <u>Radical Remission</u> emphasizes the need to be the lead decision-maker.[5] You should feel empowered to search for books or articles about your treatment using PubMed and other cancer sites mentioned in this book. You should also feel confident in asking your oncologist for books or articles as well as an explanation

> You are the owner and operator of your body.

that can help you understand the rationale behind the proposed treatment. You are the owner and operator of your body and you want your oncologist to respect you as an active participant in your healing.

❖❖❖❖❖❖❖❖❖❖❖❖❖❖❖❖❖
Notes and Questions
❖❖❖❖❖❖❖❖❖❖❖❖❖❖❖❖❖

Epilogue

In prior chapters, I have mentioned phases of the cancer journey that I took with my mom. Two years after her diagnosis, she began to develop persistent swelling in both lower legs and feet. The swelling made her legs feel heavy and made it harder to wear her shoes. The physician administering her vitamin C infusions found that her potassium was low and ordered potassium tablets to try to reduce the swelling. She began to worry about how her ski season would go if she couldn't get her feet into her ski boots. Nevertheless, she sent my brother out with her skis to get them sharpened. Her Christmas list contained other items for her life including a new pickleball paddle. She apparently was wearing out her other paddle through her vicious dropshot. She also asked for a learn-to-crochet kit as she was to resume chemo with the drug Gemzar. Her cancer had progressed and the palliative radiation that was on the table in the summer was off the table by October. Mom was discouraged, primarily because the oncologist had let a resident break the news about her cancer progression rather than telling her himself. A relationship that had been built on mutual trust was eroded in her eyes - she felt her oncologist had given up on her. My mom had an opinion at MD Anderson in New Jersey and felt the physician there was a good backup should her concerns remain.

While my mom didn't have quite the same level of energy due to difficulty walking with swollen legs, she was determined to have a great set of holidays. My brother and his wife had my parents over for Thanksgiving and my kids and I helped her prep for Christmas dinner. My mom also conceded it was perhaps too much to have her one brother and his family on Christmas and we all agreed to a get-together with deli sandwiches a few days after the holidays. We could be together, just in a different way.

In the first week of the new year, my mom and I boarded a plane to Boston. She needed wheelchair transport because her legs were so swollen, but my mom was excited to get an opinion by Jennifer's oncologist at Dana Farber. We arrived at our hotel and we had lunch. Mom laid down to rest and I did some grading. That evening we had dinner and my mom even had a glass of wine. We laughed at her persistent inability to pronounce Pinot Noir correctly.

The next day, the appointment was amazing. I found myself wishing that my mom had agreed to see the oncologist the previous summer. The genetic counselor met with us, went over my mom's prior genetic testing and decided she should have additional testing to pursue other markers that had not been tested. She felt the initial testing was appropriate, but also wanted to leave no stone unturned should a new medication become available. We then met with the oncologist who put my mom right at ease. He agreed with the high dose vitamin C infusions my mom was getting, but suggested she try the ALA infusions again. This could help her reduce her blood sugar level that was creeping slightly higher as her pancreas function became more compromised, which in turn would provide less fuel for cancer cells to divide. He felt a slower infusion might allow her to tolerate the ALA better. He was concerned about her lower body weight and suggested that she try to snack throughout the day to give her enough fuel to continue to fight the cancer. His other recommendation was to have a drain placed in her lung. My mom had already had her lung drained once, but he felt that until the therapy he was going to recommend worked, that this would be easier; a nurse could come to the home to drain it if needed.

Most importantly, he noted that her cancer tumor molecular profiling showed that her tumor had a BRCA2 mutation. A new drug Lynparza had been approved the prior week for the treatment of pancreas cancers with BRCA mutations. Lynparza was a targeted therapy in pill form. He also felt this was why my mom achieved no evidence of disease status the prior year when she was on oxaliplatin, as BRCA mutations are platinum-therapy sensitive. He suggested 1-2 months of oxaliplatin infusions with the 5-FU infused by the pump over 48 hours versus the bolus that she had switched to the prior time she had therapy. He stated that this was to help reduce her risk of infection. These 1-2 months would be followed by the Lynparza. My mom and I left that appointment elated.

The next week, we went to her regular oncologist who did not agree with the assessment of the use of Lynparza. He felt it would only be useful in germline BRCA mutations, which are the heritable mutations and not in tumor BRCA mutations. My research found this statement to be incorrect. He agreed to do it but was not enthusiastic. He was adamant on the bolus of 5-FU instead of the infusion pump. I told my mom we could do one round of this, but that we would either get the Dana Farber doctor involved or switch to the MD Anderson doctor. If worst came to worst, we would go to Boston every other week for a few days.

At the end of January, my mom had to go to the emergency department for a health issue the home health nurse was concerned about - we never did find out what the concern was. My mom picked up an infection at the hospital. She came home, but she really wasn't doing well. Several of her ALA infusions had to be canceled. One Saturday, she woke up in the middle of the night with a high fever. She tried to call to my father but wasn't sure if she was actually calling out loud or if he didn't hear her. By that morning she was delirious, and my dad called an ambulance. My brother met them at the hospital where they began to test for the source of the infection. By the time I got to the hospital in the early afternoon, she had no confusion and was admitted to the intensive care unit for observation and IV antibiotics.

The physicians could not find where the infection was coming from, but my mom continued to rally on Sunday. On Monday, her oncologist was talking about hospice care with no rationale given. When my brother and I arrived, my mom was fully lucid and using her expansive vocabulary. She was concerned that we had some decisions to make. By 10:00 that evening, my mom was unconscious and intubated. She never regained consciousness and passed away surrounded by her entire family telling her stories and sending her love.

In the early days after her death, I second guessed every decision we made. Did the bolus of 5-FU make her more susceptible to that unknown infection? Should I have pushed her oncologist harder the previous summer to resume the oxaliplatin? This was stopped at one point because mom had a rash that may have been a reaction to the chemotherapy. Should I have insisted on seeing the Dana Farber doctor earlier? Later, I wondered if perhaps she was an early case of Covid-19 that began to be identified in the few weeks after her death – the first case in our county was identified in the hospital where she had been.

In the end however, I have come to see my mom's cancer journey as somewhat miraculous. She was diagnosed in November of

2017 and had two good years of travel, pickleball and skiing. She continued to help me homeschool both of my daughters and planned so many fun activities for them to do together. She had three birthdays and Christmases and two Thanksgivings that were not guaranteed. I believe firmly that by taking charge of her own health and pairing traditional cancer treatment approaches with supplements, holistic treatments, nutrition, and exercise that she had over two years of good quality of life and joy in the face of a cancer prognosis with a 6- to 11-month median survival rate.[1]

While my mom's story ultimately ends, yours is just beginning. I hope that what we learned during our cancer journey will help you make more informed decisions and take control of your health and treatment. I wish you success on your journey.

Additional Resources

This is a compilation of media that I found helpful during my mom's cancer treatment. Because my mom did not follow a Keto diet, I do not have a recipe book recommendation for this way of eating.

Books and Essays

Ball S. *The 30-minute Mediterranean Diet Cookbook: 101 Easy, Flavorful Recipes for Lifelong Health.* Emeryville, CA: Rockridge Press; 2018.

- This is a great first-timer's cookbook for following the Mediterranean diet.

Carr K. *Crazy, Sexy Cancer Tips.* Guilford, CT.: Skirt!; 2007.

- This book gives advice from Carr's and other's cancer journeys.

Carr K. *Crazy Sexy Diet: Eat Your Veggies, Ignite Your Spark, and Live Like You Mean It!* Guilford, CT: Skirt!; 2011.

- This book provides nutrition advice for a vegetarian diet of whole and raw foods.

Centeno N. *Soup Cleanse Cookbook.* New York, NY: Rodale; 2016.

- This cookbook is full of soothing vegetarian soups that was an easy way to get vegetables into my mom when she wasn't feeling great from chemo.

Esselstyn AC, Esselstyn J. *The Prevent and Reverse Heart Disease Cookbook.* New York, NY: Avery; 2014.

- This cookbook is grounded in a whole food, plant-based diet.

Gould SJ. The median isn't the message. Virtual Mentor. 2013;15:77-81. doi: 10.1001/virtualmentor.2013.15.1.mnar1-1301. https://journalofethics.ama-assn.org/article/median-isnt-message/2013-01

- I love this essay both because of the writer and my love of statistics. I fell in love with Stephen Jay Gould's writing on evolutionary biology when I was in college. This is an essay that he wrote when he was diagnosed with cancer in the 1980s. His message is one that provides hope and reminds us that survival statistics don't represent all people with cancer. They didn't represent my mom. Strive to be an outlier.

Li WW. *Eat to Beat Disease.* New York: Grand Central Publishing; 2019.

- This book provides a thorough discussion of the healing power of foods to fight diseases including cancer.

McClelland J. *How to Starve Cancer: Without Starving Yourself.* London: Agenor Publishing; 2018:404.

- McClelland is a UK-based physiotherapist who was diagnosed with stage IV cancer. She did research to help stop her cancer from growing and ended up achieving no evidence of disease. Her transit map of blocking the different pathways of fat, protein, and sugar that cancer cells use as fuel to survive and divide is comprehensive and would be great to discuss with an integrative or functional medicine doctor. Her approach is similar to that used by the Care Oncology Clinic.

Michalsen A. *The Nature Cure.* New York, NY.: Viking; 2019.

- Dr. Michalsen is a physician and a professor of clinical complementary medicine at a university in Berlin, Germany. His insights into natural approaches to treating disease are well-researched.

Servan-Schreiber D. *Anticancer: A New Way of Life.* New York: Penguin Books; 2017.

- Dr. Servan-Schreiber describes how his own cancer diagnosis led him to understand how our health can be influenced by our lifestyle, environment, and even trauma we may experience.

Turner KA. *Radical Remission: Surviving Cancer against All Odds.* 2nd ed. New York: HarperCollins; 2014:1-313.

- Dr. Turner began this book while completing her PhD because she realized that no one was studying people who experienced an unexplained cancer remission. This book covers nine factors common to people who experience radical remission.

Turner KA. *Radical Hope: 10 Key Healing Factors from Exceptional Survivors of Cancer and Other Diseases.* Carslbad, CA: Hay House, Inc.; 2020.

- This book was published while I completed my own book. Turner adds a 10th factor, exercise, to her keys to radical remission and each chapter tells the story of a radical remission that illustrates one of the 10 factors of unexplained disease remission.

Wark C. *Chris Beat Cancer: A Comprehensive Plan for Healing Naturally.* 2nd ed. Carlsbad, CA: Hay House, Inc.; 2021.

- Wark discusses his path away from conventional cancer treatment to one of holistic healing. While I am a firm believer in a combined approach of both conventional and holistic treatments, his story is inspiring and sparked a good conversation between my mom and I about her nutrition.

DVD

Carr K. *Crazy Sexy Cancer.* [DVD]. Gaiam - Entertainment; 2008.

- This is a documentary made by Carr after she was diagnosed as having Stage IV of a rare form of cancer. Because there was no treatment for her cancer, she documents her interviews with various holistic practitioners.

Acknowledgements

This book would not have been possible without support from my family and friends, who cheer me on in all of my endeavors. I particularly want to thank my colleague and friend Dr. Dawn Gulick, who proofread multiple times, offered design ideas, and with a quiet place to write in her home. Thank you also to Dr. Jeremy Sutton, who provided a forum to encourage and assist writers in generating a book concept and taking these concepts to publication.

References

Chapter 1 References

1. Berkson BM, Calvo Riera F. The long-term survival of a patient with stage IV renal cell carcinoma following an integrative treatment approach including the intravenous alpha-lipoic Acid/Low-dose naltrexone protocol. *Integr Cancer Ther*. 2018;17(3):986-993.

2. Berkson BM, Rubin DM, Berkson AJ. Revisiting the ALA/N (alpha-lipoic acid/low-dose naltrexone) protocol for people with metastatic and nonmetastatic pancreatic cancer: A report of 3 new cases. *Integr Cancer Ther*. 2009;8(4):416-422.

3. Berkson BM, Rubin DM, Berkson AJ. The long-term survival of a patient with pancreatic cancer with metastases to the liver after treatment with the intravenous alpha-lipoic acid/low-dose naltrexone protocol. *Integr Cancer Ther*. 2006;5(1):83-89.

Chapter 2 References

1. Moss R. Moss reports. https://www.mossreports.com/. Updated 2019. Accessed 11/14, 2020.

2. Berkson BM, Calvo Riera F. The long-term survival of a patient with stage IV renal cell carcinoma following an integrative treatment approach including the intravenous alpha-lipoic Acid/Low-dose naltrexone protocol. *Integr Cancer Ther*. 2018;17(3):986-993.

3. Berkson BM, Rubin DM, Berkson AJ. Revisiting the ALA/N (alpha-lipoic acid/low-dose naltrexone) protocol for people with metastatic and nonmetastatic pancreatic cancer: A report of 3 new cases. *Integr Cancer Ther*. 2009;8(4):416-422.

4. Berkson BM, Rubin DM, Berkson AJ. The long-term survival of a patient with pancreatic cancer with metastases to the liver after treatment with the intravenous alpha-lipoic acid/low-dose naltrexone protocol. *Integr Cancer Ther.* 2006;5(1):83-89.

5. Turner K. Embracing social support. In: *Radical remission: Surviving cancer against all odds.* New York: HarperCollins Publishers; 2014:193-216.

6. Kroenke CH. A conceptual model of social networks and mechanisms of cancer mortality, and potential strategies to improve survival. *Transl Behav Med.* 2018;8(4):629-642.

7. Kroenke CH, Michael YL, Poole EM, et al. Postdiagnosis social networks and breast cancer mortality in the after breast cancer pooling project. *Cancer.* 2017;123(7):1228-1237.

8. Vogt TM, Mullooly JP, Ernst D, Pope CR, Hollis JF. Social networks as predictors of ischemic heart disease, cancer, stroke and hypertension: Incidence, survival and mortality. *J Clin Epidemiol.* 1992;45(6):659-666.

9. Cairo Notari S, Favez N, Notari L, Charvoz L, Delaloye JF. The caregiver burden in male romantic partners of women with non-metastatic breast cancer: The protective role of couple satisfaction. *J Health Psychol.* 2017;22(13):1668-1677.

10. Muscatell KA, Eisenberger NI, Dutcher JM, Cole SW, Bower JE. Links between inflammation, amygdala reactivity, and social support in breast cancer survivors. *Brain Behav Immun.* 2016;53:34-38.

11. Li MY, Yang YL, Liu L, Wang L. Effects of social support, hope and resilience on quality of life among Chinese bladder cancer patients: A cross-sectional study. *Health Qual Life Outcomes*. 2016;14:73-016-0481-z.

12. Haviland J, Sodergren S, Calman L, et al. Social support following diagnosis and treatment for colorectal cancer and associations with health-related quality of life: Results from the UK ColoREctal wellbeing (CREW) cohort study. *Psychooncology*. 2017;26(12):2276-2284.

13. Gonzalez-Saenz de Tejada M, Bilbao A, Bare M, et al. Association between social support, functional status, and change in health-related quality of life and changes in anxiety and depression in colorectal cancer patients. *Psychooncology*. 2017;26(9):1263-1269.

14. An E, Lo C, Hales S, Zimmermann C, Rodin G. Demoralization and death anxiety in advanced cancer. *Psychooncology*. 2018;27(11):2566-2572.

15. De Padova S, Casadei C, Berardi A, et al. Caregiver emotional burden in testicular cancer patients: From patient to caregiver support. *Front Endocrinol (Lausanne)*. 2019;10:318.
16. Dionne-Odom JN, Hull JG, Martin MY, et al. Associations between advanced cancer patients' survival and family caregiver presence and burden. *Cancer Med*. 2016;5(5):853-862.

17. Tang ST, Chen JS, Chou WC, et al. Prevalence of severe depressive symptoms increases as death approaches and is associated with disease burden, tangible social support, and high self-perceived burden to others. *Support Care Cancer*. 2016;24(1):83-91.

18. Admiraal JM, van Nuenen FM, Burgerhof JG, Reyners AK, Hoekstra-Weebers JE. Cancer patients' referral wish: Effects of distress, problems, socio-demographic and illness-related variables and social support sufficiency. *Psychooncology.* 2016;25(11):1363-1370.

19. Drageset S, Lindstrom TC, Giske T, Underlid K. Women's experiences of social support during the first year following primary breast cancer surgery. *Scand J Caring Sci.* 2016;30(2):340-348.

20. Manne SL, Kashy DA, Virtue S, et al. Acceptance, social support, benefit-finding, and depression in women with gynecological cancer. *Qual Life Res.* 2018;27(11):2991-3002.

21. Banik A, Luszczynska A, Pawlowska I, Cieslak R, Knoll N, Scholz U. Enabling, not cultivating: Received social support and self-efficacy explain quality of life after lung cancer surgery. *Ann Behav Med.* 2017;51(1):1-12.

22. Dennis CL. Peer support within a health care context: A concept analysis. *Int J Nurs Stud.* 2003;40(3):321-332.

23. Holt-Lunstad J, Smith TB, Layton JB. Social relationships and mortality risk: A meta-analytic review. *PLoS Med.* 2011;7:e1000316.

24. Salakari M, Pylkkanen L, Sillanmaki L, et al. Social support and breast cancer: A comparatory study of breast cancer survivors, women with mental depression, women with hypertension and healthy female controls. *Breast.* 2017;35:85-90.

25. Fleisch Marcus A, Illescas AH, Hohl BC, Llanos AA. Relationships between social isolation, neighborhood poverty, and cancer mortality in a population-based study of US adults. *PLoS One.* 2017;12(3):e0173370.

26. Wu Z, Nguyen NH, Wang D, et al. Social connectedness and mortality after prostate cancer diagnosis: A prospective cohort study. *Int J Cancer*. 2019.

27. Koch-Gallenkamp L, Bertram H, Eberle A, et al. Fear of recurrence in long-term cancer survivors-do cancer type, sex, time since diagnosis, and social support matter? *Health Psychol*. 2016;35(12):1329-1333.

28. Thompson T, Perez M, Kreuter M, Margenthaler J, Colditz G, Jeffe DB. Perceived social support in African American breast cancer patients: Predictors and effects. *Soc Sci Med*. 2017;192:134-142.

29. Fong AJ, Scarapicchia TMF, McDonough MH, Wrosch C, Sabiston CM. Changes in social support predict emotional well-being in breast cancer survivors. *Psychooncology*. 2017;26(5):664-671.

30. Nausheen B, Gidron Y, Peveler R, Moss-Morris R. Social support and cancer progression: A systematic review. *J Psychosom Res*. 2009;67(5):403-415.

31. Merluzzi TV, Philip EJ, Yang M, Heitzmann CA. Matching of received social support with need for support in adjusting to cancer and cancer survivorship. *Psychooncology*. 2016;25(6):684-690.

32. Jan M, Bonn SE, Sjolander A, et al. The roles of stress and social support in prostate cancer mortality. *Scand J Urol*. 2016;50(1):47-55.

33. Gage-Bouchard EA, LaValley S, Mollica M, Beaupin LK. Communication and exchange of specialized health-related support among people with experiential similarity on facebook. *Health Commun*. 2017;32(10):1233-1240.

34. Gage-Bouchard EA, LaValley S, Mollica M, Beaupin LK. Cancer communication on social media: Examining how cancer caregivers use Facebook for cancer-related communication. *Cancer Nurs.* 2017;40(4):332-338.

35. Zhang S, O'Carroll Bantum E, Owen J, Bakken S, Elhadad N. Online cancer communities as informatics intervention for social support: Conceptualization, characterization, and impact. *J Am Med Inform Assoc.* 2017;24(2):451-459.

36. Belong app. Belong app website. https://belong.life/. Accessed 11/14, 2020.

37. Parker Oliver D, Patil S, Benson JJ, et al. The effect of internet group support for caregivers on social support, self-efficacy, and caregiver burden: A meta-analysis. *Telemed J E Health.* 2017;23(8):621-629.

38. Burnette D, Duci V, Dhembo E. Psychological distress, social support, and quality of life among cancer caregivers in albania. *Psychooncology.* 2017;26(6):779-786.

39. Halpern MT, Fiero MH, Bell ML. Impact of caregiver activities and social supports on multidimensional caregiver burden: Analyses from nationally-representative surveys of cancer patients and their caregivers. *Qual Life Res.* 2017;26(6):1587-1595.

40. Krieger JL. Family communication about cancer treatment decision-making. In: Cohen E, ed. *Communication yearbook.* New York: Routledge; 2014:279-305.

41. Krok-Schoen JL, Palmer-Wackerly AL, Dailey PM, Wojno JC, Krieger JL. Age differences in cancer treatment decision making and social support. *J Aging Health.* 2017;29(2):187-205.

Chapter 3 References

1. American Cancer Society. Cancer staging. www.cancer.org Website. https://www.cancer.org/treatment/understanding-your-diagnosis/staging.html. Published 03/25/2015. Updated 2015. Accessed 04/09, 2020.

2. American Society of Clinical Oncology. Stages of cancer. www.cancer.net Website. https://www.cancer.net/navigating-cancer-care/diagnosing-cancer/stages-cancer. Published 03/2018. Updated 2018. Accessed 04/09, 2020.

3. American Society of Clinical Oncology. Understanding your complete bood count (CBC) tests. https://www.cancer.net/navigating-cancer-care/diagnosing-cancer/reports-and-results/understanding-your-complete-blood-count-cbc-tests. Published 06/2019. Updated 2019. Accessed 04/16, 2020.

4. American Society of Clinical Oncology. Tumor marker tests. www cancer.net Website. https://www.cancer.net/navigating-cancer-care/diagnosing-cancer/tests-and-procedures/tumor-marker-tests. Published 05/2018. Updated 2018. Accessed 04/16, 2020.

5. National Cancer Institute. Tumor markers in common use. https://www.cancer.gov/about-cancer/diagnosis-staging/diagnosis/tumor-markers-list. Updated 2019. Accessed 11/17, 2020.

6. American Cancer Society. Types of biopsies to look for cancer. www.cancer.org Website. https://www.cancer.org/treatment/understanding-your-diagnosis/tests/testing-biopsy-and-cytology-specimens-for-cancer/biopsy-types.html. Published 07/30/2015. Updated 2015. Accessed 04/09, 2020.

7. Robson ME, Bradbury AR, Arun B, et al. American society of clinical oncology policy statement update: Genetic and genomic testing for cancer susceptibility. *J Clin Oncol*. 2015;33(31):3660-3667.

8. El-Deiry WS, Goldberg RM, Lenz HJ, et al. The current state of molecular testing in the treatment of patients with solid tumors, 2019. *CA Cancer J Clin*. 2019;69(4):305-343.

9. Foundation Medicine. What is FoundationOne CDx? FoundationOne CDx Website. https://www.startwithstepone.com/. Published 2019. Updated 2019. Accessed 11/18, 2020.

10. American Cancer Society. CT scan for cancer. cancer.org Website. https://www.cancer.org/treatment/understanding-your-diagnosis/tests/ct-scan-for-cancer.html. Published 11/30/2015. Updated 2015. Accessed 04/09, 2020.

11. Griffeth LK. Use of PET/CT scanning in cancer patients: Technical and practical considerations. *Proc (Bayl Univ Med Cent)*. 2005;18(4):321-330.

12. American Cancer Society. Tubes, lines, ports and catheters used in cancer treatment. cancer.org Website. https://www.cancer.org/treatment/treatments-and-side-effects/planning-managing/tubes-lines-ports-catheters.html. Published 02/11/2016. Updated 2020. Accessed 11/15, 2020.

13. American Cancer Society. How is chemotherapy used to treat cancer? cancer.org Website. https://www.cancer.org/treatment/treatments-and-side-effects/treatment-types/chemotherapy/how-is-chemotherapy-used-to-treat-cancer.html. Published 11/22/2019. Updated 2019. Accessed 04/07, 2020.

14. DeVita VT,Jr. Chu E. A history of cancer chemotherapy. *Cancer Res*. 2008;68(21):8643-8653.

15. Oken MM, Creech RH, Tormey DC, et al. Toxicity and response criteria of the Eastern Cooperative Oncology Group. *Am J Clin Oncol*. 1982;5(6):649-655.

16. American Cancer Society. Chemotherapy side effects. cancer.org Website. https://www.cancer.org/treatment/treatments-and-side-effects/treatment-types/chemotherapy/chemotherapy-side-effects.html. Published 11/22/2019. Updated 2019. Accessed 04/07, 2020.

17. Romiti A, Cox MC, Sarcina I, et al. Metronomic chemotherapy for cancer treatment: A decade of clinical studies. *Cancer Chemother Pharmacol*. 2013;72(1):13-33.

18. Baskar R, Lee KA, Yeo R, Yeoh KW. Cancer and radiation therapy: Current advances and future directions. *Int J Med Sci*. 2012;9(3):193-199.

19. Demaria S, Golden EB, Formenti SC. Role of local radiation therapy in cancer immunotherapy. *JAMA Oncol*. 2015;1(9):1325-1332.

20. National Cancer Institute. Surgery to treat cancer. www.cancer.gov Website. https://www.cancer.gov/about-cancer/treatment/types/surgery. Published 4/29/2015. Updated 2015. Accessed 04/16, 2020.

21. American Cancer Society. Stem cell transplant. www.cancer.org Website. https://www.cancer.org/treatment/treatments-and-side-effects/treatment-types/stem-cell-transplant/donors.html. Accessed 02/06, 2021.

22. Jourabchi N, Beroukhim K, Tafti BA, Kee ST, Lee EW. Irreversible electroporation (NanoKnife) in cancer treatment. *Gastrointestinal Intervention.* 2014;3(1):8-18.

23. Lee YT, Tan YJ, Oon CE. Molecular targeted therapy: Treating cancer with specificity. *Eur J Pharmacol.* 2018;834:188-196.

24. American Society of Clinical Oncology. Understanding immunotherapy. www.cancer.net Website. https://www.cancer.net/navigating-cancer-care/how-cancer-treated/immunotherapy-and-vaccines/understanding-immunotherapy. Published 01/2019. Updated 2019. Accessed 04/2020, 2020.

25. Koo SL, Wang WW, Toh HC. Cancer immunotherapy - the target is precisely on the cancer and also not. *Ann Acad Med Singapore.* 2018;47(9):381-387.

26. Yelamos J, Galindo M, Navarro J, et al. Enhancing tumor-targeting monoclonal antibodies therapy by PARP inhibitors. *Oncoimmunology.* 2015;5(1):e1065370.

27. American Cancer Society. What are the phases of clinical trials? American Cancer Society Website. https://www.cancer.org/treatment/treatments-and-side-effects/clinical-trials/what-you-need-to-know/phases-of-clinical-trials.html. Published 05/03/2016. Updated 2017. Accessed 04/20, 2020.

28. Jarrow JP, Lurie P, Ikenberry SC, Lemery S. Overview of FDA's expanded access program for investigational drugs. *Ther Innov Regul Sci.* 2017;51(1):177-179.

29. Center for Information and Study of Clinical Research Participation. Find a trial. www.ciscrp.org Website. https://www.ciscrp.org/services/search-clinical-trials/search-trials-now/. Updated 2020. Accessed 04/20, 2020.

30. National Cancer Institute. Find NCI-supported clinical trials. www.cancer.gov Website. https://www.cancer.gov/about-cancer/treatment/clinical-trials/search. Accessed 04/20, 2020.

31. National Institute of Health. Clinical trials. https://www.clinicaltrials.gov/. Published 5/7/2020. Updated 2020. Accessed 11/19, 2020.

32. PanCan. Clinical trials. Pancreatic Cancer Action Network Website. https://www.pancan.org/facing-pancreatic-cancer/treatment/treatment-types/clinical-trials/. Published 2020. Updated 2020. Accessed 11/17, 2020.

33. National Library of Medicine. PubMed. https://pubmed.ncbi.nlm.nih.gov/. Published 2020. Updated 2020. Accessed 11/19, 2020.

34. Turner KA. *Radical remission: Surviving cancer against all odds.* 2nd ed. New York: HarperCollins; 2014:1-313.

Chapter 4 References

1. Drageset S, Lindstrom TC, Giske T, Underlid K. Women's experiences of social support during the first year following primary breast cancer surgery. *Scand J Caring Sci.* 2016;30(2):340-348.

2. Turner K. Taking control of your health. In: *Radical remission: Surviving cancer against all odds.* New York: HarperCollins Publishers; 2014:45-74.

3. American Society of Clinical Oncology. Types of oncologists https://www.cancer.net/navigating-cancer-care/cancer-basics/cancer-care-team/types-oncologists#:~:text=An%20oncologist%20is%20a%20do

ctor,as%20targeted%20therapy%20or%20immunotherapy
. Published 2020. Updated 2020. Accessed 11/18, 2020.

4. American Occupational Therapy Association. About
occupational therapy. American Occupational Therapy
Association Website. https://www.aota.org/About-
Occupational-Therapy/Patients-Clients.aspx. Published
2020. Updated 2020. Accessed 11/18, 2020.

5. Cancer Care. The value of oncology social workers.
https://www.cancercare.org/publications/262-
the_value_of_oncology_social_workers. Published 2020.
Updated 2020. Accessed 11/19, 2020.

6. American Physical Therapy Association. Find a PT.
Choose PT Website.
https://aptaapps.apta.org/APTAPTDirectory/FindAPTDir
ectory.aspx. Published 2019. Updated 2019. Accessed
2020, 11/18.

7. American Psychological Association. What is cognitive
behavioral therapy? Clinical practice guideline for the
treatment of post-traumatic stress disorder.Website.
https://www.apa.org/ptsd-guideline/patients-and-
families/cognitive-behavioral. Published 2017. Updated
2020. Accessed 11/18, 2020.

8. Garland SN, Xie SX, DuHamel K, et al. Acupuncture
versus cognitive behavioral therapy for insomnia in
cancer survivors: A randomized clinical trial. *J Natl
Cancer Inst*. 2019;111(12):1323-1331.

9. Kucherer S, Ferguson RJ. Cognitive behavioral therapy
for cancer-related cognitive dysfunction. *Curr Opin
Support Palliat Care*. 2017;11(1):46-51.

10. Sandler CX, Goldstein D, Horsfield S, et al.
Randomized evaluation of cognitive-behavioral therapy
and graded exercise therapy for post-cancer fatigue. *J
Pain Symptom Manage*. 2017;54(1):74-84.

11. Feros DL, Lane L, Ciarrochi J, Blackledge JT. Acceptance and commitment therapy (ACT) for improving the lives of cancer patients: A preliminary study. *Psychooncology*. 2013;22(2):459-464.

12. Wolfram T. Nutrition during and after cancer treatment. Academy of Nutrition and Dietetics Website. https://www.eatright.org/health/diseases-and-conditions/cancer/nutrition-during-and-after-cancer-treatment. Published 6/29/2017. Updated 2017. Accessed 11/19, 2020.

13. Academy of Nutrition and Dietetics. Find an expert. 2020. Updated 2020. Accessed 11/19, 2020.

14. American Association for Respiratory Care. What RTs do. https://be-an-rt.org/what-is-respiratory-therapy/what-rts-do/. Published 2020. Updated 2020. Accessed 11/18, 2020.

15. American Speech Language Hearing Association. About the CSD professions: Speech-language pathology. https://www.asha.org/students/speech-language-pathology/#:~:text=Speech%2Dlanguage%20pathologists%20(SLPs),disorders%20in%20children%20and%20adults. Published 2020. Updated 2020. Accessed 11/18, 2020.

16. Buss MK, Rock LK, McCarthy EP. Understanding palliative care and hospice: A review for primary care providers. *Mayo Clin Proc*. 2017;92(2):280-286.

17. National Hospice and Palliative Care Organization. Patients and caregivers. https://www.nhpco.org/patients-and-caregivers/. Published 2020. Updated 2020. Accessed 11/18, 2020.

Chapter 5 References

1. Fuchs T, Hanaya H, Seilacher E, et al. Information deficits and second opinion seeking - A survey on cancer patients. *Cancer Invest.* 2017;35(1):62-69.

2. Kurian AW, Friese CR, Bondarenko I, et al. Second opinions from medical oncologists for early-stage breast cancer: Prevalence, correlates, and consequences. *JAMA Oncol.* 2017;3(3):391-397.

3. Radhakrishnan A, Grande D, Mitra N, Bekelman J, Stillson C, Pollack CE. Second opinions from urologists for prostate cancer: Who gets them, why, and their link to treatment. *Cancer.* 2017;123(6):1027-1034.

4. Ruetters D, Keinki C, Schroth S, Liebl P, Huebner J. Is there evidence for a better health care for cancer patients after a second opinion? A systematic review. *J Cancer Res Clin Oncol.* 2016;142(7):1521-1528.

5. Tattersall MH, Dear RF, Jansen J, et al. Second opinions in oncology: The experiences of patients attending the sydney cancer centre. *Med J Aust.* 2009;191(4):209-212.

6. Hillen MA, Medendorp NM, Daams JG, Smets EMA. Patient-driven second opinions in oncology: A systematic review. *Oncologist.* 2017;22(10):1197-1211.

7. Garcia D, Spruill LS, Irshad A, Wood J, Kepecs D, Klauber-DeMore N. The value of a second opinion for breast cancer patients referred to a national cancer institute (NCI)-designated cancer center with a multidisciplinary breast tumor board. *Ann Surg Oncol.* 2018;25(10):2953-2957.

8. Grevenkamp F, Kommoss F, Kommoss F, et al. Second opinion expert pathology in endometrial cancer: Potential clinical implications. *Int J Gynecol Cancer.* 2017;27(2):289-296.

9. Heeg E, Civil YA, Hillen MA, et al. Impact of second opinions in breast cancer diagnostics and treatment: A retrospective analysis. *Ann Surg Oncol.* 2019;26(13):4355-4363.

10. Tosteson ANA, Yang Q, Nelson HD, et al. Second opinion strategies in breast pathology: A decision analysis addressing over-treatment, under-treatment, and care costs. *Breast Cancer Res Treat.* 2018;167(1):195-203.

11. Lineback CM, Mervak CM, Revels SL, Kemp MT, Reddy RM. Barriers to accessing optimal esophageal cancer care for socioeconomically disadvantaged patients. *Ann Thorac Surg.* 2017;103(2):416-421.

12. Haider M. Why second opinions matter - my father's journey from
suffering with cancer to living with it. *Cancer Research Statistics and Treatment.* 2019;2(2):169-171.

Chapter 6 References

1. Samuels N, Freed Y, Weitzen R, et al. Feasibility of homeopathic treatment for symptom reduction in an integrative oncology service. *Integr Cancer Ther.* 2018;17(2):486-492.

2. Danno K, Colas A, Freyer G, et al. Motivations of patients seeking supportive care for cancer from physicians prescribing homeopathic or conventional medicines: Results of an observational cross-sectional study. *Homeopathy.* 2016;105(4):289-298.

3. Fulop JA, Grimone A, Victorson D. Restoring balance for people with cancer through integrative oncology. *Prim Care*. 2017;44(2):323-335.

4. Jermini M, Dubois J, Rodondi PY, et al. Complementary medicine use during cancer treatment and potential herb-drug interactions from a cross-sectional study in an academic centre. *Sci Rep*. 2019;9(1):5078-019-41532-3.

5. Schuerger N, Klein E, Hapfelmeier A, Kiechle M, Brambs C, Paepke D. Evaluating the demand for integrative medicine practices in breast and gynecological cancer patients. *Breast Care (Basel)*. 2019;14(1):35-40.

6. Gras M, Vallard A, Brosse C, et al. Use of complementary and alternative medicines among cancer patients: A single-center study. *Oncology*. 2019;97(1):18-25.

7. Frenkel M. Is there a role for homeopathy in cancer care? questions and challenges. *Curr Oncol Rep*. 2015;17(9):43-015-0467-8.

8. Kacel EL, Pereira DB, Estores IM. Advancing supportive oncology care via collaboration between psycho-oncology and integrative medicine. *Support Care Cancer*. 2019;27(9):3175-3178.

9. Stub T, Quandt SA, Arcury TA, et al. Perception of risk and communication among conventional and complementary health care providers involving cancer patients' use of complementary therapies: A literature review. *BMC Complement Altern Med*. 2016;16:353-016-1326-3.

10. Stub T, Quandt SA, Arcury TA, Sandberg JC, Kristoffersen AE. Conventional and complementary cancer treatments: Where do conventional and complementary providers seek information about these

184

modalities? *BMC Health Serv Res*. 2018;18(1):854-018-3674-9.

11. Frenkel M, Ben-Arye E, Cohen L. Communication in cancer care: Discussing complementary and alternative medicine *Integr Cancer Ther*. 2010;9(2):177-185.

12. Moss R. Moss reports. https://www.mossreports.com/. Updated 2019. Accessed 11/14, 2020.

13. Amer can Association of Naturopathic Physicians. What is a naturopathic doctor? https://naturopathic.org/page/WhatisaNaturopathicDoctor. Accessed 12/1, 2020.

14. Psihogios A, Ennis JK, Seely D. Naturopathic oncology care for pediatric cancers: A practice survey. *Integr Cancer Ther*. 2019;18:1534735419878504.
15. American Association of Naturopathic Physicians. Find a doctor. https://naturopathic.org/search/custom.asp?id=5613. Accessed 12/1, 2020.

16. McClelland J. *How to starve cancer: Without starving yourself*. London: Agenor Publishing; 2018:404.

17. Care Oncology Clinic. Care oncology-schedule initial consultation. https://careoncology.com/products/initial-consult-pre-pay/. Accessed 12/2, 2020.

18. Care Oncology Clinic. Faq. https://careoncology.com/faq/. Accessed 12/2, 2020.

19. Focused Ultrasound Foundation. For patients. https://www.fusfoundation.org/for-patients/how-it-works. Updated 2020. Accessed 12/10, 2020.

20. Focused Ultrasound Foundation. Treatment sites. https://www.fusfoundation.org/the-technology/treatment-sites. Updated 2020. Accessed 12/10, 2020.

21. Berkson BM, Calvo Riera F. The long-term survival of a patient with stage IV renal cell carcinoma following an integrative treatment approach including the intravenous alpha-lipoic Acid/Low-dose naltrexone protocol. *Integr Cancer Ther*. 2018;17(3):986-993.

22. Berkson BM, Rubin DM, Berkson AJ. Revisiting the ALA/N (alpha-lipoic acid/low-dose naltrexone) protocol for people with metastatic and nonmetastatic pancreatic cancer: A report of 3 new cases. *Integr Cancer Ther*. 2009;8(4):416-422.

23. Berkson BM, Rubin DM, Berkson AJ. Reversal of signs and symptoms of a B-cell lymphoma in a patient using only low-dose naltrexone. *Integr Cancer Ther*. 2007;6(3):293-296.

24. Berkson BM, Rubin DM, Berkson AJ. The long-term survival of a patient with pancreatic cancer with metastases to the liver after treatment with the intravenous alpha-lipoic acid/low-dose naltrexone protocol. *Integr Cancer Ther*. 2006;5(1):83-89.

25. Nauman G, Gray JC, Parkinson R, Levine M, Paller CJ. Systematic review of intravenous ascorbate in cancer clinical trials. *Antioxidants (Basel)*. 2018;7(7):10.3390/antiox7070089.

26. Deng G, Cassileth B. Complementary or alternative medicine in cancer care-myths and realities. *Nat Rev Clin Oncol*. 2013;10(11):656-664.

27. Pellati F, Borgonetti V, Brighenti V, Biagi M, Benvenuti S, Corsi L. Cannabis sativa L. and nonpsychoactive cannabinoids: Their chemistry and role against oxidative stress, inflammation, and cancer. *Biomed Res Int*. 2018;2018:1691428.

28. Sledzinski P, Zeyland J, Slomski R, Nowak A. The current state and future perspectives of cannabinoids in cancer biology. *Cancer Med*. 2018;7(3):765-775.

29. Jeon SM, Shin EA. Exploring vitamin D metabolism and function in cancer. *Exp Mol Med*. 2018;50(4):20-018-0038-9.
30. Minisola S, Ferrone F, Danese V, et al. Controversies surrounding vitamin D: Focus on supplementation and cancer. *Int J Environ Res Public Health*. 2019;16(2):10.3390/ijerph16020189.

31. Mondul AM, Weinstein SJ, Layne TM, Albanes D. Vitamin D and cancer risk and mortality: State of the science, gaps, and challenges. *Epidemiol Rev*. 2017;39(1):28-48.

32. Zhang Y, Fang F, Tang J, et al. Association between vitamin D supplementation and mortality: Systematic review and meta-analysis. *BMJ*. 2019;366:l4673.

33. Grant WB. Review of recent advances in understanding the role of vitamin D in reducing cancer risk: Breast, colorectal, prostate, and overall cancer. *Anticancer Res*. 2020;40(1):491-499.

34. Goulao B, Stewart F, Ford JA, MacLennan G, Avenell A. Cancer and vitamin D supplementation: A systematic review and meta-analysis. *Am J Clin Nutr*. 2018;107(4):652-663.

35. Talib WH. Melatonin and cancer hallmarks. *Molecules*. 2018;23(3):10.3390/molecules23030518.

36. Li Y, Li S, Zhou Y, et al. Melatonin for the prevention and treatment of cancer. *Oncotarget*. 2017;8(24):39896-39921.

37. Reiter RJ, Rosales-Corral SA, Tan DX, et al. Melatonin, a full service anti-cancer agent: Inhibition of initiation, progression and metastasis. *Int J Mol Sci.* 2017;18(4):10.3390/ijms18040843.

38. Farhood B, Goradel NH, Mortezaee K, Khanlarkhani N, Najafi M, Sahebkar A. Melatonin and cancer: From the promotion of genomic stability to use in cancer treatment. *J Cell Physiol.* 2019;234(5):5613-5627.

39. Boon H, Wong J. Botanical medicine and cancer: A review of the safety and efficacy. *Expert Opin Pharmacother.* 2004;5(12):2485-2501.

40. PDQ Integrative, Alternative, and Complementary Therapies Editorial Board. Medicinal mushrooms (PDQ(R)): Health professional version. In: *PDQ cancer information summaries.* Bethesda (MD); 2002. NBK401261 [bookaccession].

41. Leonard SS, Keil D, Mehlman T, Proper S, Shi X, Harris GK. Essiac tea: Scavenging of reactive oxygen species and effects on DNA damage. *J Ethnopharmacol.* 2006;103(2):288-296.

42. Tamayo C, Richardson MA, Diamond S, Skoda I. The chemistry and biological activity of herbs used in flor-essence herbal tonic and essiac. *Phytother Res.* 2000;14(1):1-14.

43. Kaegi E. Unconventional therapies for cancer: 1. Essiac. the task force on alternative therapies of the canadian breast cancer research initiative. *CMAJ.* 1998;158(7):897-902.

44. Ottenweller J, Putt K, Blumenthal EJ, Dhawale S, Dhawale SW. Inhibition of prostate cancer-cell proliferation by essiac. *J Altern Complement Med.* 2004;10(4):687-691.

45. Al-Sukhni W, Grunbaum A, Fleshner N. Remission of hormone-refractory prostate cancer attributed to Essiac. *Can J Urol*. 2005;12(5):2841-2842.

46. Shirakami Y, Shimizu M. Possible mechanisms of green tea and its constituents against cancer. *Molecules*. 2018;23(9):10.3390/molecules23092284.

47. Ohishi T, Goto S, Monira P, Isemura M, Nakamura Y. Anti-inflammatory action of green tea. *Antiinflamm Antiallergy Agents Med Chem*. 2016;15(2):74-90.

48. Liossi C. Hypnosis in cancer care. *Contemporary Hypnosis*. 2006;23(1):47-57.

49. National Certification Commission for Acupuncture and Oriental Medicine. Find a practitioner. https://directory.nccaom.org/. Accessed 12/1, 2020.

50. Sagar SM, Dryden T, Wong RK. Massage therapy for cancer patients: A reciprocal relationship between body and mind. *Curr Oncol*. 2007;14(2):45-56.

51. Boyd C, Crawford C, Paat CF, et al. The impact of massage therapy on function in pain populations-A systematic review and meta-analysis of randomized controlled trials: Part II, cancer pain populations. *Pain Med*. 2016;17(8):1553-1568.

52. Noh GO, Park KS. Effects of aroma self-foot reflexology on peripheral neuropathy, peripheral skin temperature, anxiety, and depression in gynaecologic cancer patients undergoing chemotherapy: A randomised controlled trial. *Eur J Oncol Nurs*. 2019;42:82-89.

53. Rambod M, Pasyar N, Shamsadini M. The effect of foot reflexology on fatigue, pain, and sleep quality in lymphoma patients: A clinical trial. *Eur J Oncol Nurs*. 2019;43:101678.

54. Lymphology Association of North America. Find a LANA-certified therapist. https://www.clt-lana.org/search/therapists/. Updated 2020. Accessed 2020, 11/21.

55. Rao RM, Amritanshu R, Vinutha HT, et al. Role of yoga in cancer patients: Expectations, benefits, and risks: A review. *Indian J Palliat Care.* 2017;23(3):225-230.

56. Wayne PM, Lee MS, Novakowski J, et al. Tai chi and qigong for cancer-related symptoms and quality of life: A systematic review and meta-analysis. *J Cancer Surviv.* 2018;12(2):256-267.

57. Lundt A, Jentschke E. Long-term changes of symptoms of anxiety, depression, and fatigue in cancer patients 6 months after the end of yoga therapy. *Integr Cancer Ther.* 2019;18:1534735418822096.

58. Lin PJ, Kleckner IR, Loh KP, et al. Influence of yoga on cancer-related fatigue and on mediational relationships between changes in sleep and cancer-related fatigue: A nationwide, multicenter randomized controlled trial of yoga in cancer survivors. *Integr Cancer Ther.* 2019;18:1534735419855134.

59. Cramer H, Lauche R, Klose P, Lange S, Langhorst J, Dobos GJ. Yoga for improving health-related quality of life, mental health and cancer-related symptoms in women diagnosed with breast cancer. *Cochrane Database Syst Rev.* 2017;1:CD010802.

60. yoga4cancer. https://y4c.com/. Updated 2021. Accessed 01/01, 2021.

61. Reis D, Jones T. Aromatherapy: Using essential oils as a supportive therapy. *Clin J Oncol Nurs.* 2017;21(1):16-19.

Chapter 7 References

1. Kerr J, Anderson C, Lippman SM. Physical activity, sedentary behaviour, diet, and cancer: An update and emerging new evidence. *Lancet Oncol*. 2017;18(8):e457-e471.

2. Cormie P, Trevaskis M, Thornton-Benko E, Zopf EM. Exercise medicine in cancer care. *Aust J Gen Pract*. 2020;49(4):169-174.

3. American Heart Association. Physical activity. https://www.heart.org/en/get-involved/advocate/federal-priorities/physical-activity. Published 2018. Updated 2018. Accessed 2020, 11/22.

4. Lobelo F, Rohm Young D, Sallis R, et al. Routine assessment and promotion of physical activity in healthcare settings: A scientific statement from the american heart association. *Circulation*. 2018;137(18):e495-e522.

5. Vainshelboim B, Lima RM, Myers J. Cardiorespiratory fitness and cancer in women: A prospective pilot study. *J Sport Health Sci*. 2019;8(5):457-462.

6. Weiderpass E. Lifestyle and cancer risk. *J Prev Med Public Health*. 2010;43(6):459-471.

7. U.S. Department of Health and Human Services, ed. *Physical activity guidelines for all americans,* 2nd. ed. Washington, D.C.: U.S. Department of Health and Human Services; 2018.

8. Schwartz AL, de Heer HD, Bea JW. Initiating exercise interventions to promote wellness in cancer patients and survivors. *Oncology (Williston Park)*. 2017;31(10):711-717.

9. Stout NL, Baima J, Swisher AK, Winters-Stone KM, Welsh J. A systematic review of exercise systematic reviews in the cancer literature (2005-2017). *PM R.* 2017;9(9S2):S347-S384.

10. Reed JL, Pipe AL. The talk test: A useful tool for prescribing and monitoring exercise intensity. *Curr Opin Cardiol.* 2014;29(5):475-480.

11. Stoggl TL, Sperlich B. The training intensity distribution among well-trained and elite endurance athletes. *Front Physiol.* 2015;6:295.

12. Borg G. *Borg's perceived exertion and pain scales.* Champaign, IL: Human Kinetics; 1998.

13. American College of Sports Medicine. Exercise prescription for healthy populations with special considerations. In: Riebe D, Ehrman JK, Liguori G, Magal M, eds. *Guidelines for exercise testing and prescription.* 10th ed. Philadelphia, PA: Wolters Kluwer; 2018:180-208.

14. Idorn M, Thor Straten P. Exercise and cancer: From "healthy" to "therapeutic"? *Cancer Immunol Immunother.* 2017;66(5):667-671.

15. Brown JC, Harhay MO, Harhay MN. Physical function as a prognostic biomarker among cancer survivors. *Br J Cancer.* 2015;112(1):194-198.

16. McTiernan A, Friedenreich CM, Katzmarzyk PT, et al. Physical activity in cancer prevention and survival: A systematic review. *Med Sci Sports Exerc.* 2019;51(6):1252-1261.

17. Wennerberg E, Lhuillier C, Rybstein MD, et al. Exercise reduces immune suppression and breast cancer progression in a preclinical model. *Oncotarget.* 2020;11(4):452-461.

18. Sitlinger A, Brander DM, Bartlett DB. Impact of exercise on the immune system and outcomes in hematologic malignancies. *Blood Adv*. 2020;4(8):1801-1811.

19. Sheill G, Guinan E, O'Neill L, et al. Preoperative exercise to improve fitness in patients undergoing complex surgery for cancer of the lung or oesophagus (PRE-HIIT): Protocol for a randomized controlled trial. *BMC Cancer*. 2020;20(1):321-020-06795-4.

20. An KY, Kang DW, Morielli AR, et al. Patterns and predictors of exercise behavior during 24 months of follow-up after a supervised exercise program during breast cancer chemotherapy. *Int J Behav Nutr Phys Act*. 2020;17(1):23-020-00924-9.

21. Guida JL, Agurs-Collins T, Ahles TA, et al. Strategies to prevent or remediate cancer and treatment-related aging. *J Natl Cancer Inst*. 2020.
22. Sebio Garcia R, Yanez Brage MI, Gimenez Moolhuyzen E, Granger CL, Denehy L. Functional and postoperative outcomes after preoperative exercise training in patients with lung cancer: A systematic review and meta-analysis. *Interact Cardiovasc Thorac Surg*. 2016;23(3):486-497.

23. Edbrooke L, Granger CL, Denehy L. Physical activity for people with lung cancer. *Aust J Gen Pract*. 2020;49(4):175-181.

24. Kesting S, Weeber P, Schonfelder M, Renz BW, Wackerhage H, von Luettichau I. Exercise as a potential intervention to modulate cancer outcomes in children and adults? *Front Oncol.* 2020;10:196.

25. Brown JC, Winters-Stone K, Lee A, Schmitz KH. Cancer, physical activity, and exercise. *Compr Physiol.* 2012;2(4):2775-2809.

26. Del-Rosal-Jurado A, Romero-Galisteo R, Trinidad-Fernandez M, Gonzalez-Sanchez M, Cuesta-Vargas A, Ruiz-Munoz M. Therapeutic physical exercise post-treatment in breast cancer: A systematic review of clinical practice guidelines. *J Clin Med.* 2020;9(4):10.3390/jcm9041239.

27. Mascherini G, Ringressi MN, Castizo-Olier J, et al. Preliminary results of an exercise program after laparoscopic resective colorectal cancer surgery in non-metastatic adenocarcinoma: A pilot study of a randomized control trial. *Medicina (Kaunas).* 2020;56(2):10.3390/medicina56020078.

28. Wiggenraad F, Bolam KA, Mijwel S, van der Wall E, Wengstrom Y, Altena R. Long-term favorable effects of physical exercise on burdensome symptoms in the OptiTrain breast cancer randomized controlled trial. *Integr Cancer Ther.* 2020;19:1534735420905003.

29. Chang PH, Lin CR, Lee YH, et al. Exercise experiences in patients with metastatic lung cancer: A qualitative approach. *PLoS One.* 2020;15(4):e0230188.

30. Ulrich CM, Himbert C, Holowatyj AN, Hursting SD. Energy balance and gastrointestinal cancer: Risk, interventions, outcomes and mechanisms. *Nat Rev Gastroenterol Hepatol.* 2018;15(11):683-698.

31. Fonseca GWPD, Farkas J, Dora E, von Haehling S, Lainscak M. Cancer cachexia and related metabolic dysfunction. *Int J Mol Sci*. 2020;21(7):10.3390/ijms21072321.

32. Jain R, Handorf E, Khare V, Blau M, Chertock Y, Hall MJ. Impact of baseline nutrition and exercise status on toxicity and outcomes in phase I and II oncology clinical trial participants. *Oncologist*. 2020;25(2):161-169.

33. McDonald L, Oguz M, Carroll R, et al. Comparison of accelerometer-derived physical activity levels between individuals with and without cancer: A UK biobank study. *Future Oncol*. 2019;15(33):3763-3774.

34. Friedenreich CM, Stone CR, Cheung WY, Hayes SC. Physical activity and mortality in cancer survivors: A systematic review and meta-analysis. *JNCI Cancer Spectr*. 2019;4(1):pkz080.

35. Jung AY, Behrens S, Schmidt M, et al. Pre- to postdiagnosis leisure-time physical activity and prognosis in postmenopausal breast cancer survivors. *Breast Cancer Res*. 2019;21(1):117-019-1206-0.

36. Schmitz KH, Courneya KS, Matthews C, et al. American college of sports medicine roundtable on exercise guidelines for cancer survivors. *Med Sci Sports Exerc*. 2010;42(7):1409-1426.

37. Kraschnewski JL, Sciamanna CN, Poger JM, et al. Is strength training associated with mortality benefits? A 15year cohort study of US older adults. *Prev Med*. 2016;87:121-127.

38. Cheville AL, Mustian K, Winters-Stone K, Zucker DS, Gamble GL, Alfano CM. Cancer rehabilitation: An overview of current need, delivery models, and levels of care. *Phys Med Rehabil Clin N Am*. 2017;28(1):1-17.

39. Stout NL, Silver JK, Raj VS, et al. Toward a national initiative in cancer rehabilitation: Recommendations from a subject matter expert group. *Arch Phys Med Rehabil.* 2016;97(11):2006-2015.

40. Nicol JL, Woodrow C, Burton NW, et al. Physical activity in people with multiple myeloma: Associated factors and exercise program preferences. *J Clin Med.* 2020;9(10):10.3390/jcm9103277.

41. Haussmann A, Gabrian M, Ungar N, et al. What hinders healthcare professionals in promoting physical activity towards cancer patients? the influencing role of healthcare professionals' concerns, perceived patient characteristics and perceived structural factors. *Eur J Cancer Care (Engl).* 2018;27(4):e12853.

42. Lopez G, Eddy C, Liu W, et al. Physical therapist-led exercise assessment and counseling in integrative cancer care: Effects on patient self-reported symptoms and quality of life. *Integr Cancer Ther.* 2019;18:1534735419832360.

43. Rey Lopez JP, Gebel K, Chia D, Stamatakis E. Associations of vigorous physical activity with all-cause, cardiovascular and cancer mortality among 64 913 adults. *BMJ Open Sport Exerc Med.* 2019;5(1):e000596.

Chapter 8 References

1. Gorn D. Food as medicine is no longer a fringe idea. KQED Website. https://www.kqed.org/futureofyou/310438/food-as-medicine-its-not-just-a-fringe-idea-anymore. Published 01/25/2017. Updated 2017. Accessed 03/04, 2021.

2. Dinu M, Abbate R, Gensini GF, Casini A, Sofi F. Vegetarian, vegan diets and multiple health outcomes: A systematic review with meta-analysis of observational studies. *Crit Rev Food Sci Nutr*. 2017;57(17):3640-3649.

3. Aune D, Giovannucci E, Boffetta P, et al. Fruit and vegetable intake and the risk of cardiovascular disease, total cancer and all-cause mortality-a systematic review and dose-response meta-analysis of prospective studies. *Int J Epidemiol*. 2017;46(3):1029-1056.

4. Chen J, Campbell TC, Li J, Peto R. *Diet, life-style and mortality in China: A study of the characteristics of 65 Chinese counties.*. Oxford, UK: Oxford University Press; 1990.

5. Chlebowski RT, Blackburn GL, Thomson CA, et al. Dietary fat reduction and breast cancer outcome: Interim efficacy results from the women's intervention nutrition study. *J Natl Cancer Inst*. 2006;98(24):1767-1776.

6. Ocvirk S, Wilson AS, Appolonia CN, Thomas TK, O'Keefe SJD. Fiber, fat, and colorectal cancer: New insight into modifiable dietary risk factors. *Curr Gastroenterol Rep*. 2019;21(11):62-019-0725-2.

7. Qi XX, Shen P. Associations of dietary protein intake with all-cause, cardiovascular disease, and cancer mortality: A systematic review and meta-analysis of cohort studies. *Nutr Metab Cardiovasc Dis*. 2020;30(7):1094-1105.

8. Fung TT, van Dam RM, Hankinson SE, Stampfer M, Willett WC, Hu FB. Low-carbohydrate diets and all-cause and cause-specific mortality: Two cohort studies. *Ann Intern Med*. 2010;153(5):289-298.

9. Yin J, Ren W, Huang X, Li T, Yin Y. Protein restriction and cancer. *Biochim Biophys Acta Rev Cancer*. 2018;1869(2):256-262.

10. Campbell TC. Cancer prevention and treatment by wholistic nutrition. *J Nat Sci*. 2017;3(10).

11. McCarty MF. Vegan proteins may reduce risk of cancer, obesity, and cardiovascular disease by promoting increased glucagon activity. *Med Hypotheses*. 1999;53(6):459-485.

12. Levine ME, Suarez JA, Brandhorst S, et al. Low protein intake is associated with a major reduction in IGF-1, cancer, and overall mortality in the 65 and younger but not older population. *Cell Metab*. 2014;19(3):407-417.

13. Papier K, Tong TY, Appleby PN, et al. Comparison of major protein-source foods and other food groups in meat-eaters and non-meat-eaters in the EPIC-oxford cohort. *Nutrients*. 2019;11(4):10.3390/nu11040824.

14. Brandhorst S, Longo VD. Protein quantity and source, fasting-mimicking diets, and longevity. *Adv Nutr*. 2019;10(Suppl_4):S340-S350.

15. Campbell TC. Nutritional renaissance and public health policy. *J Nutr Biol*. 2017;3(1):124-138.

16. Ornish D, Lin J, Chan JM, et al. Effect of comprehensive lifestyle changes on telomerase activity and telomere length in men with biopsy-proven low-risk prostate cancer: 5-year follow-up of a descriptive pilot study. *Lancet Oncol*. 2013;14(11):1112-1120.

17. Ornish D, Magbanua MJ, Weidner G, et al. Changes in prostate gene expression in men undergoing an intensive nutrition and lifestyle intervention. *Proc Natl Acad Sci U S A*. 2008;105(24):8369-8374.

18. Ornish D, Magbanua MJ, Weidner G, et al. Changes in prostate gene expression in men undergoing an intensive nutrition and lifestyle intervention. *Proc Natl Acad Sci U S A*. 2008;105(24):8369-8374.

19. Orman A, Johnson DL, Comander A, Brockton N. Breast cancer: A lifestyle medicine approach. *Am J Lifestyle Med*. 2020;14(5):483-494.

20. Tuttolomondo A, Simonetta I, Daidone M, Mogavero A, Ortello A, Pinto A. Metabolic and vascular effect of the Mediterranean diet. *Int J Mol Sci*. 2019;20(19):10.3390/ijms20194716.

21. Vicinanza R, Troisi G, Cangemi R, et al. Aging and adherence to the Mediterranean diet: Relationship with cardiometabolic disorders and polypharmacy. *J Nutr Health Aging*. 2018;22(1):73-81.

22. Eleftheriou D, Benetou V, Trichopoulou A, La Vecchia C, Bamia C. Mediterranean diet and its components in relation to all-cause mortality: Meta-analysis. *Br J Nutr*. 2018;120(10):1081-1097.

23. Morze J, Danielewicz A, Przybylowicz K, Zeng H, Hoffmann G, Schwingshackl L. An updated systematic review and meta-analysis on adherence to Mediterranean diet and risk of cancer. *Eur J Nutr*. 2020.

24. Tosti V, Bertozzi B, Fontana L. Health benefits of the Mediterranean diet: Metabolic and molecular mechanisms. *J Gerontol A Biol Sci Med Sci*. 2018;73(3):318-326.

25. Di Daniele N, Noce A, Vidiri MF, et al. Impact of Mediterranean diet on metabolic syndrome, cancer and longevity. *Oncotarget*. 2017;8(5):8947-8979.

26. Newman TM, Vitolins MZ, Cook KL. From the table to the tumor: The role of Mediterranean and western dietary patterns in shifting microbial-mediated signaling to impact breast cancer risk. *Nutrients*. 2019;11(11):10.3390/nu11112565.

27. Ostan R, Lanzarini C, Pini E, et al. Inflammaging and cancer: A challenge for the Mediterranean diet. *Nutrients*. 2015;7(4):2589-2621.

28. Oliviero F, Spinella P, Fiocco U, Ramonda R, Sfriso P, Punzi L. How the Mediterranean diet and some of its components modulate inflammatory pathways in arthritis. *Swiss Med Wkly*. 2015;145:w14190.

29. Henriquez Sanchez P, Ruano C, de Irala J, Ruiz-Canela M, Martinez-Gonzalez MA, Sanchez-Villegas A. Adherence to the Mediterranean diet and quality of life in the SUN project. *Eur J Clin Nutr*. 2012;66(3):360-368.

30. Silva R, Pizato N, da Mata F, Figueiredo A, Ito M, Pereira MG. Mediterranean diet and musculoskeletal-functional outcomes in community-dwelling older people: A systematic review and meta-analysis. *J Nutr Health Aging*. 2018;22(6):655-663.

31. Silva TRD, Martins CC, Ferreira LL, Spritzer PM. Mediterranean diet is associated with bone mineral density and muscle mass in postmenopausal women. *Climacteric*. 2019;22(2):162-168.

32. Rivas A, Romero A, Mariscal-Arcas M, et al. Mediterranean diet and bone mineral density in two age groups of women. *Int J Food Sci Nutr*. 2013;64(2):155-161.

33. Baguley BJ, Skinner TL, Jenkins DG, Wright ORL. Mediterranean-style dietary pattern improves cancer-related fatigue and quality of life in men with prostate cancer treated with androgen deprivation therapy: A pilot randomised control trial. *Clin Nutr*. 2021;40(1):245-254.

34. Allen BG, Bhatia SK, Anderson CM, et al. Ketogenic diets as an adjuvant cancer therapy: History and potential mechanism. *Redox Biol*. 2014;2:963-970.

35. Weber DD, Aminzadeh-Gohari S, Tulipan J, Catalano L, Feichtinger RG, Kofler B. Ketogenic diet in the treatment of cancer - where do we stand? *Mol Metab*. 2020;33:102-121.

36. Upton J. Keto v. mediterranean: Which diet is really better for you? Explore Health Website. https://www.health.com/nutrition/keto-mediterranean-diet. Published 01/28/2020. Updated 2020. Accessed 02/17, 2021.

37. Zhuang Y, Chan DK, Haugrud AB, Miskimins WK. Mechanisms by which low glucose enhances the cytotoxicity of metformin to cancer cells both in vitro and in vivo. *PLoS One*. 2014;9(9):e108444.

38. Husain Z, Huang Y, Seth P, Sukhatme VP. Tumor-derived lactate modifies antitumor immune response: Effect on myeloid-derived suppressor cells and NK cells. *J Immunol*. 2013;191(3):1486-1495.

39. Aminzadeh-Gohari S, Feichtinger RG, Vidali S, et al. A ketogenic diet supplemented with medium-chain triglycerides enhances the anti-tumor and anti-angiogenic efficacy of chemotherapy on neuroblastoma xenografts in a CD1-nu mouse model. *Oncotarget*. 2017;8(39):64728-64744.

40. Stafford P, Abdelwahab MG, Kim DY, Preul MC, Rho JM, Scheck AC. The ketogenic diet reverses gene expression patterns and reduces reactive oxygen species levels when used as an adjuvant therapy for glioma. *Nutr Metab (Lond)*. 2010;7:74-7075-7-74.

41. Klement RJ. The emerging role of ketogenic diets in cancer treatment. *Curr Opin Clin Nutr Metab Care*. 2019;22(2):129-134.

42. Mattson MP, Longo VD, Harvie M. Impact of intermittent fasting on health and disease processes. *Ageing Res Rev*. 2017;39:46-58.

43. Wei M, Brandhorst S, Shelehchi M, et al. Fasting-mimicking diet and markers/risk factors for aging, diabetes, cancer, and cardiovascular disease. *Sci Transl Med*. 2017;9(377):10.1126/scitranslmed.aai8700.

44. Antunes F, Erustes AG, Costa AJ, et al. Autophagy and intermittent fasting: The connection for cancer therapy? *Clinics (Sao Paulo)*. 2018;73(suppl 1):e814s.

45. Brandhorst S, Longo VD. Fasting and caloric restriction in cancer prevention and treatment. *Recent Results Cancer Res*. 2016;207:241-266.

46. Lee-Kwan SH, Moore LV, Blanck HM, Harris DM, Galuska D. Disparities in state-specific adult fruit and vegetable consumption - united states, 2015. *MMWR*. 2017;66(45):1241-1247.

47. Serafini M, Peluso I. Functional foods for health: The interrelated antioxidant and anti-inflammatory role of fruits, vegetables, herbs, spices and cocoa in humans. *Curr Pharm Des*. 2016;22(44):6701-6715.

48. Johnson RK, Appel LJ, Brands M, et al. Dietary sugars intake and cardiovascular health: A scientific statement from the American Heart Association. *Circulation*. 2009;120(11):1011-1020.

Chapter 9 References

1. Rocque GB, Rasool A, Williams BR, et al. What is important when making treatment decisions in metastatic breast cancer? A qualitative analysis of decision-making in patients and oncologists. *Oncologist*. 2019;24(10):1313-1321.

2. Gidwani-Marszowski R, Nevedal AL, Blayney DW, et al. Oncologists' views on using value to guide cancer treatment decisions. *Value Health*. 2018;21(8):931-937.

3. Patient Access Network Foundation. https://www.panfoundation.org/. Published 2020. Updated 2020. Accessed 11/19, 2020.

4. Truglio-Londrigan M, Slyer JT, Singleton JK, Worral P. A qualitative systematic review of internal and external influences on shared decision-making in all health care settings. *JBI Libr Syst Rev*. 2012;10(58):4633-4646.

5. Turner K. Taking control of your health. In: *Radical remission: Surviving cancer against all odds.* New York: HarperCollins Publishers; 2014:45-74.

Epilogue Reference

1. Pancreatic cancer-survival. Cancer Research UK Website. https://www.cancerresearchuk.org/about-cancer/pancreatic-cancer/survival. Published 09/26/2019. Updated 2019. Accessed 11/15, 2020.

www.ingramcontent.com/pod-product-compliance
Lightning Source LLC
Chambersburg PA
CBHW041214030426
42336CB00023B/3339